TALK **SEX** TODAY

Wow! This book surpassed all my expectations ... I learned so much about talking to my children about sexual health, and I laughed out loud more times than I can count! Saleema has such a gift for delivering material many of us – including myself – find awkward in a humorous, accessible and thoughtful way. Covering everything from the scientific facts to gender identity to Internet exposure to appearance pressures and so much more. I truly believe this is the only book parents will ever need to educate themselves and their kids on sexual health. I know I'll be referring to it for many years to come.
– Cea Sunrise Person, bestselling author of *North of Normal*

As a journalist I have often relied on Saleema Noon's expertise when we cover stories about sexual health. As a parent, I'm grateful for this inclusive, relatable book to help me answer those tough questions my kids are starting to ask. Sexual health is not an easy subject for everyone – Saleema's book *Talk Sex Today* is inclusive and real, making it easy for all of us to have authentic conversations about our bodies.
– Tamara Taggart, OBC, CTV News Anchor

Those of us who take sex ed to the schools know that it can be both risky business and lots of fun. Our communities are diverse in terms of religious beliefs, ethno-cultural backgrounds and attitudes towards sex. Balancing the dangers of unsafe sex and sexualized violence with the pleasurable aspects of sex is important. As sex educators we don't want to turn kids off sex because it's too dangerous, yet we hope that whenever they engage in sexual activity, it's from a positive and empowered place. Following in the footsteps of Meg Hickling, Saleema Noon is well known for teaching children and youth about sex in accessible and enlightening ways. This book is teeming with valuable information about sexual health (or body science as the author calls it). Celebrated in BC for her candid and accessible sexuality education, Saleema Noon has done a fine job of writing about the work she had done with young people of various ages, teaching them about sexuality in a positive way, as opposed to the fear-based methods often used by adults. The book lays out a general curriculum for appropriate information about sexuality for different ages. It includes sections on kids with special needs, managing the Internet, sexualized violence and other important topics. It's an easy read and one that would be helpful for parents, teachers and others who wish to learn how to talk about sex with young people. Take a peek!
– Dr. Farah Shroff, Faculty Member, Department of Family Practice and School of Population and Public Health

TalkSex

SALEEMA NOON AND MEG HICKLING

Today

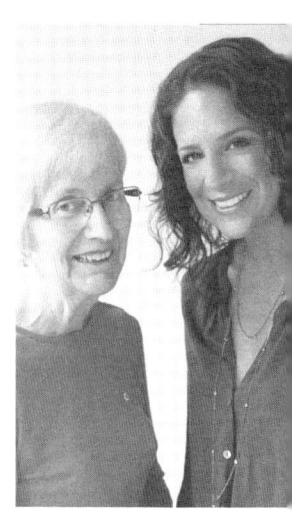

WHAT KIDS NEED TO KNOW AND HOW ADULTS CAN TEACH THEM

WOOD LAKE

Editor: Mike Schwartzentruber
Designer: Robert MacDonald

Library and Archives Canada Cataloguing in Publication
Noon, Saleema, 1971-, author
Talk sex today : what kids need to know and how adults can teach them / Saleema Noon and Meg Hickling.
Includes bibliographical references and index.
Issued in print and electronic formats.
ISBN 978-1-77064-813-5 (paperback).—ISBN 978-1-77064-814-2 (html)
1. Sex instruction for children. I. Hickling, Meg, 1941-, author II. Title.
HQ53.N66 2016   649'.65   C2016-904066-6   C2016-904067-4

Copyright © 2016 Saleema Noon and Meg Hickling
All rights reserved. No part of this publication may be reproduced – except in the case of brief quotations embodied in critical articles and reviews – stored in an electronic retrieval system, or transmitted in any form or by any means, electronic, mechanical, photocopying, recording, or otherwise, without prior written permission of the publisher or copyright holder.

ISBN 978-1-77064-813-5

Published by Wood Lake Publishing Inc.
485 Beaver Lake Road, Kelowna, BC, Canada, V4V 1S5
www.woodlake.com | 250.766.2778

We acknowledge the financial support of the Government of Canada. Nous reconnaissons l'appui financier du gouvernement du Canada. Wood Lake Publishing acknowledges the financial support of the Province of British Columbia through the Book Publishing Tax Credit.

At Wood Lake Publishing, we practice what we publish, being guided by a concern for fairness, justice, and equal opportunity in all of our relationships with employees and customers. Wood Lake Publishing is committed to caring for the environment and all creation. Wood Lake Publishing recycles and reuses, and encourages readers to do the same. Books are printed on 100% post-consumer recycled paper, whenever possible. A percentage of all profit is donated to charitable organizations.

Printed in Canada by Friesens
Printing 10 9 8 7 6 5 4 3 2 1

TABLE OF CONTENTS

Preface 8
Introduction 9

1. **Talk Sex Today** 19
2. **Gender and Sexuality** 31
   Creating a Common Language
3. **The Magical Thinkers** 45
   Preschoolers (Preschool–Grade 1)
4. **The Bathroom Humour Types** 75
   Primaries (Grades 2–3)
5. **The Gross-Me-Outers** 95
   Intermediates (Grades 4–5)
6. **Managing Media and the Internet** 135
   Intermediates (Grades 4–5)
7. **Managing Media and the Internet** 153
   Intermediates (Grades 6–7)
8. **Sexual Consent and Gender Stereotypes** ... 175
   Intermediates (Grades 6–7)
9. **Relationships, Sex, and Health** 191
   Intermediates (Grades 6–7)
10. **Relationships and Healthy Boundaries** 219
    Adolescents (Grades 8–12)
11. **Sex Talk? No Sweat** 239
    Adolescents (Grades 8–12)
12. **Straight Answers to Sticky Questions** 271
13. **Teaching Sexual Health to Children and Teens with Special Needs** 289

Conclusion:
From Body Science to Sexually Mature Adult 309
Index 313

DEDICATIONS

SALEEMA NOON

To my husband, Chris, who has been a staunch supporter of the work I do from the moment I met him, and who has demonstrated beautifully the value of honest, open conversations between a dad and his daughters. Not only has he waited countless times for me to get home from teaching at night so that we can have dinner together, but he's tolerated me and my laptop parked at the kitchen island for the past year and a half as I've written this revised and expanded book.

MEG HICKLING

I'd like to dedicate this edition to my husband, Tony, who cheerfully accepts and replies to emails on my behalf. His support has meant everything to me in this work.

ACKNOWLEDGEMENTS

I'd like to thank Meg Hickling for taking a chance on me fresh out of graduate school, for teaching me how to teach, for trusting me to carry on her legacy and to write a new edition of her book, for continuing to be a mentor and a friend, and for showing me what life-long commitment to making change looks like.

I'd like to thank my stepdaughters, Afton and Kate, who were always proud to have me teach at their schools, who've trusted me to answer even the "most awkward" questions, and who have given me permission to share dozens of their personal body science adventures with others in my teaching.

I'd like to thank my makeup-artist sister and best friend, Alisha Noon. She's the only person I know who can create the perfect brow while at the same time convince the parent in her chair that I could save their child's life by visiting their school. Plus, she has done my makeup for dozens of photos and TV interviews over the years.

Thank you also my to parents, who not only put me through eight years of university, but who have supported me wholeheartedly in my career, life, and literally everything I do.

Thank you to my extraordinary team of educators: Brandy Wiebe, Ashley McIntosh, Anna Soole, Cath Blythe, Brandon Burke, and Ryan Avola. To say that I've learned so much from each one of them doesn't even begin to cover it. They're just as committed to our work as I am; they've brought our workshops to a level I could have never imagined, and I'm in awe when I see them in action. Extra love to Cath who, in addition to teaching, has taken on the massive role of keeping us all organized so that I could devote the time needed to write this revised and expanded book. Huge gratitude also to Brandy for lending her eagle eyes and super smarts to my manuscript in its final stages.

And thank you to Mike Schwartzentruber, my editor at Wood Lake Publishing, for feeling totally comfortable sending me emails with subject lines such as "labia etc.," for his skill in making my jumbled thoughts sound really good, and for being an absolute pleasure to work with in general.

Last but not least, Meg and I would both like to acknowledge the thousands of students we've taught over the years. Teachers and parents have come to our workshops with open minds and have trusted us to send meaningful, positive messages to their kids. Children and teens have reminded us every day that they're capable of understanding so much more than we think, that curiosity is something to be nurtured, and that we're actually pretty funny. We'll watch with pride as these young people lead the way toward a sexually mature society for generations to come.

Saleema Noon

PREFACE

People have often asked me how I got started teaching parents how to talk with their children about sexual health issues. I think my passion for educating children and their parents arose from my nursing experience. I was appalled by my patients' lack of knowledge about their bodies and their sexual health. Sometimes that lack of knowledge resulted in very serious consequences, even death. I was determined to teach my own children about their bodies in their preschool years. Of course, they took that knowledge into the community and soon other parents began asking how they could make their own children as comfortable and as knowledgeable as mine.

I began teaching sexual health in 1974. That was the time when the "flower children" of the 1960s were beginning parents. They were more open to hearing their children's questions, but had no role models to follow. Parents of previous generations had either not heard the questions, or had ignored them, or had given erroneous answers. You might say that I was in the right place at the right time!

Fast-forward to the 21st century. Today, parents and children have some of the same gaps in their knowledge, but there are also totally new areas of concern, and many, many more questions. In the early 1970s there was no Internet, virtually no access to pornography (apart from *Playboy*), no cell phones, no AIDS, and no real awareness of child sexual abuse. Times have changed!

That is why I am so pleased that Saleema Noon has agreed to revise *Speaking of Sex* and its sequels. Saleema was, first, my student, and then my colleague. She is a first-rate educator. With her many talents and innovations, she has greatly extended the field well beyond the vision I had in 1974.

It is with a tremendous amount of pride that I introduce her to you. I know that you and the children in your care and sphere will be exceedingly well-cared-for as you read this book. Don't forget to laugh at Saleema's stories and even at yourself sometimes. You will learn a lot, I believe, and be much more sexually mature by the time you reach the end of the book.

Best wishes,
Meg Hickling

INTRODUCTION

As a sexual health educator, I spend most of my time teaching children, teens, parents, and those who work with kids about healthy bodies and healthy sexuality. It's something I've been doing for 18 years now, and as I tell my students, it's the best job in the world.

Over the years, Grade 4 and 5 students have asked me questions like, "Who convinced you to do this job?" and "Of all the jobs in the world you could have picked, why would you choose one as gross as this?"

I tell them that, when I was their age, I wanted to be a backup dancer for Madonna. When that didn't pan out, my Plan B was to be a teacher. But as I made my way through university and into my first "real" job, my mission became clear.

In the first term of my master's degree in family studies, I was assigned to be a teaching assistant (TA) for a third-year human sexuality class. After grading the students' first exam of the course, I was shocked at how little information these 21-year-olds had about their bodies – some of them didn't even know how many openings they had between their legs! Then for my thesis research, I interviewed 14 Grade 10 students (15-year-olds) about their sex education experience. They told me pretty much unanimously that their sex education was a joke. They ridiculed the outdated videos their teachers were forced to show them, and claimed that the information they got was stuff they already knew, while the information they *really* wanted to learn simply wasn't addressed. Overall, what they received was of very limited relevance to their lives. By the way, they volunteered to come in on a Professional Development Day off school to share this with me. Interesting.

After I graduated in 1997, I worked for two and a half years as a Family Support Worker with pregnant and parenting teens. As you can imagine, the young women I worked with (aged 14–19) taught me a lot about the value of having accurate sexual health information long before you need it. I'll never forget meeting one of my clients for the first time shortly after I started. She was 13 years old, in Grade 8, referred by her school counsellor who thought she might be pregnant. After a chat in my office, we headed to the Youth Clinic for a pregnancy test, for which the results were positive. On the drive back, she said, "Saleema, I don't get it. How is it possible that I'm pregnant? I mean, we did it on a Tuesday!" It was at that moment I realized that there was still so much work to do when it came to sexual health education.

It was around that time that I was able, through my volunteer work with Planned Parenthood Association of British Columbia (now Options for Sexual Health), to meet the legendary Meg Hickling. Although in her early 60s, she was still teaching a schedule I found difficult to contend with even in my 20s, and was looking toward retirement in a few years. She asked me to train with her and to continue teaching her "body science" programs around the province. As Oprah says, it was luck – preparation meeting opportunity. I immediately started following Meg (as well as Alice Bell, her brilliant and hilarious fellow body scientist) around to learn the ropes. And the rest is history.

My personal life has also fuelled my passion for teaching young people about sexual health. A few years after I started teaching, I met my now husband, Chris, dad to two young girls, Kate and Afton, aged five and seven at the time, respectively. As we grew closer, my drive to make sure young people had the information they needed became stronger. Teaching sexual health was no longer just about helping other people's kids stay safe, now it was personal.

Gratefully, I had permission early in our relationship not only from Chris but also from the girls' mom (Anne) to get the ball rolling with some body science discussions. It's a good thing, because after one of my first weekends spent with the girls, Kate helped herself to the sample condoms in my teaching kit that I had left in the car. Thank goodness Anne had a sense of humour when she found the condoms in Kate's pocket while doing laundry later in the week! Over the years, we've had lots of good discussions around the dinner table as a family, on the way to lessons and activities, and while watching TV together. The girls didn't always appreciate me bringing up certain topics when their friends were over, but I know that they felt proud that their stepmom, "The Sex Lady," came to teach at their schools.

Kate and Afton are now 17 and 19 years old, but when I look at the curious faces of elementary students I teach today, I see Kate and Afton in them, as the young girls I so desperately wanted to teach and protect. And I'm proud to say that today they are both well on their way to becoming sexually mature adults.

I'm happy to tell you that since Meg started her groundbreaking work in the 1970s, much has changed when it comes to how we teach body science. For instance, we rarely teach evening sessions for parents and children at elementary schools now. Rather, most of the time, parents and school administrators invite me to work with students during the school day, to ensure that *all* students (not just those whose parents bring them) benefit from life-saving body science information. Sometimes I spend a day or two with students at a school, and more and more often I'm asked to visit each classroom individually over the course of a week in order to better meet students' specific needs in a more intimate environment.

I've also noticed that, over the years, parents have become more and more supportive of the work I do with their kids. Of course, this was Meg's experience, too, but when I arrive at a school to give a presentation to parents (as I always do before working with the students) I can assume that I will be received with gratitude and support. In fact, it's rare that parents have serious doubts about what I am teaching. When they do, they ask, "Why do I have to talk to my child now, at their age? She doesn't ask questions; he's not interested; she'll be shocked; he'll be upset; she'll look at me (us) differently; I want to keep him innocent; I want them to have their childhood; they don't need to know now..."

What these parents are really saying is, "I'm not ready; I don't know what to say; I'm too embarrassed," and most of all, "I was upset when I found out and I don't want my child to be traumatized too."

There's a lot of shame in those statements, a reflection of an adult's own childhood, when information about sexuality was considered to be secret, dirty, smutty, and for adults only. Sadly, many adults carry that baggage around with them today. But there is nothing shameful about the way we make babies, and even less shame in learning about our bodies and how to take care of them. We adults need to force ourselves, force our communities, to grow up. We need to become more sexually mature to help our children. Granted, this is challenging given that most of us didn't learn from our parents about sexual health. But our children are counting on us.

Fortunately, the vast majority of parents today agree that sexual health education is crucial when it comes to keeping their kids safe and healthy. They want their children to have a better experience than they did, and they approach this education in a positive way. Never before have parents felt so empowered to start talking to their kids at an early age, and we're seeing their efforts in our Canadian statistics, when it comes to indicators like "age at first intercourse" and teen pregnancy.

> Comment: I was a little disturbed but I learned a lot.
>
> - really like how you didn't make us feel wierd and disgusted

According to the Canadian Community Health Survey done in 2009–2010, only 30% of teens aged 15 to 17 reported that they had had sexual intercourse at least once. This figure is down slightly from 1996 to 1997, when it was 32%. Statistics Canada reports that our teenage pregnancy rate has been declining steadily over the years, with 24.6 per 1000 pregnancies experienced by those under the age of 20 in 2005. If we look at the most recent decade for which we have complete data, we can see that the combined teen birth/abortion rate in Canada declined in each consecutive year, from 44.2 per 1,000 women aged 15–19 in 1996, to 27.9 in 2006, a decline of 36.9%. The Canadian teen birth rate decreased from 22.1 per 1,000 in 1996 to 14.2 in 2009 (a decline of 35.7%), and the teen abortion rate also decreased from 22.1 in 1996 to 14.2 in 2006 (a decline of 35.7%). I'm not saying that statistics are the only or best way to measure success, but we can still feel good about them!

Today, I know that I've made Meg proud by spreading her powerful message about healthy bodies and healthy sexuality. And kids and teens (although they don't often admit it) think I'm pretty cool. One time, a Grade 4 student told me that I should move to Montreal and become a comedian. Another time, a preschool student exclaimed that my body science lesson was more fun than a *Frozen* book (referring to the wildly popular Disney movie). I've been asked both by kids and adults more than once, "Do you do birthday parties?" And it always makes my day when a teen approaches me alone after class and simply thanks me for coming.

There's also never a shortage of interesting personal questions from students: "How old are you?" "What's your middle name?" "What's your favourite show?" "Do you have a boyfriend and, if not, are you married?" and my personal favourite, "Have you ever sexed before and if so did you enjoy it?"

When it comes to personal information, here are some fun facts about me that I don't mind sharing with my students:
- I don't have a middle name.
- I can tap dance.
- I have a silver lab named Jagger; he's my partner in crime.
- I love pizza. I don't love mushrooms, olives, or seafood.
- I lived in Karachi, Pakistan, for four years when I was in high school.
- I have a sister; she's my best friend.
- I've run four marathons.
- My husband, Chris, and I have the same birthday (August 10).
- I got a hole-in-one once.

Here's some information I'd like *you* to know about me:
My approach to sexual health education is sex positive and comprehensive. At every age I want kids to know that between two adults in a healthy, consenting relationship, sex is a great thing. I want them to know that it will probably be an awesome part of their lives some-

day. And sex education includes much more than just sex. It's about science, relationships, communication, health, safety, smart decision-making, and respect.

I don't believe in abstinence-only, fear-based or problem-focused sexual health education. These approaches demean young people and don't work. When we teach children and teens that sex is bad and dangerous, or when we deny their natural sexual feelings, we cause them shame, guilt, and a future of sexual problems. No thank you.

I believe that knowledge is power. We can't make smart decisions without scientific, accurate information at every age. And children are capable of understanding much more than we give them credit for.

I fiercely believe in inclusivity, that every person regardless of abilities, race, religion, age, sex, sexual attraction, romantic attraction, gen-

Is sex is good or not?

der identity or gender expression deserves respect. Our differences are something to celebrate. More specifically, I believe that every human has a right to feel safe living their truth and being who they are.

In a perfect world, parents would be their child's number one source of sexual health information, especially when it comes to teaching family values and beliefs. But I think the old saying "It takes a village" is true. We as parents, educators, relatives, close adults, role models, and professionals who work with kids need to reinforce each other's positive messages about sexuality, and work together to empower our kids.

I am beyond excited about this book and feel honoured that Meg Hickling and Wood Lake Publishing trusted me to write it. I am thrilled that you are reading it and hope that it finds a home on your night table for many years.

And finally, here's what I'd like you to know about this book so you can get the biggest bang for your buck:

This book is a joint venture between Meg and me. She's provided the foundation; she's the pioneer. Using her framework, I've brought information up to date and have expanded it to include topics and issues that have become relevant since the last edition of her book was published 10 years ago. I've added my own voice, stories and insight, based on my experience and personality.

The language I use in this book may be a different than you're used to and even cumbersome at times, particularly when it comes to gender. But there's good reason for this. Using terms like "boy," "girl," "male" and "female" works well for most people, but relying solely on them to refer to a person's gender identity excludes those who don't fit into either of the groups that we're assigned to the day we're born. And assuming that "all boys have bodies like this" or "all girls have bodies like this" is simply inaccurate. How we feel as male, female, or something entirely different is both complex and separate from how our body looks physically at birth. More on that in Chapter 2.

I use the term "parent" to include guardians or other adults who may parent, care for, and have important conversations with children, such as stepparents, foster parents, aunts, uncles and grandparents. I avoid using the terms "mom" or "dad" as they make assumptions about families that may not be accurate. (For example, sometimes it's not the mom who has the baby, and not all kids have a dad in their lives.)

Also in an effort to be inclusive, I use the term "partner" to refer to one's companion in a romantic or sexual relationship, avoiding terms like "husband," "wife," "girlfriend," or "boyfriend," which make assumptions about a relationship that may not be accurate.

I'm the first to admit that I'm not an expert on all things related to sexual health. The good news, though, is that I belong to a community of gifted educators and, together, we know pretty much everything! Just kidding. But I have drawn on their expertise in areas that aren't my specialty and, wow, are they smart.

I know you're busy. You probably don't have big chunks of time to sit down and read this book in peace. For that reason, I've written much of it in point form for quick reference. I'm hoping that you can easily take away concrete tips on specific topics as you need them.

When I work with parents, they often they ask me, "Can you just tell me again how you would explain (periods, how babies are made, what condoms are for)? I hope you find it helpful that I've written these scripts in bold font so that they stand out and can be easily referred to again and again.

Meg and I provide the Stages of Sexual Development framework simply as a guideline for parents who want to know *what* to teach their kids and *when*. These stages, and their corresponding checklists of topics to be taught, aren't rigid; they are stretchable and shrinkable.

It's never too late to provide kids with sexual health information, so please don't feel inadequate if your intermediate child only knows three things on the primary checklist. Start talking sex today and you'll be caught up in no time.

I'm writing this book as an educator, but also as a parent. Usually these two roles in my life are aligned in terms of practicing what I preach, but in the writing process I've learned that this isn't always the case (see the chapters on teenagers)!

In addition to a chapter on how to answer some tough questions that kids ask, I've also included real questions from students in the margins, to give you an idea of what children and teens are asking (and for entertainment value, of course). The answers to these questions are included in the corresponding text.

I've listed resources and tips relevant to each stage of development at the end of each chapter. My hope is that this will allow you to "grab and go."

This book doesn't present *all* the information that people need to know about healthy sexuality over their lifespan. There aren't nearly enough pages for that! Instead, I've highlighted what we know to be key topics when it comes to raising sexually healthy children and teens. There are also topics related to sexual health that, although important, I simply didn't have space to include.

This book is meant to celebrate the diversity that exists in human sexuality and the power of knowledge to create a sexually mature society for our children. I hope it paves the way for many meaningful, engaging, and fun conversations with your kids for years to come!

1. Talk Sex Today

1. Talk Sex Today

There are three reasons why it's so important that we teach our young children about sexual health – and by young I mean the day our babies are born. All of these reasons have to do with safety, prevention, and protection.

■ LITTLES MAKE THE BEST BODY SCIENTISTS

The first reason is that young children are the easiest to teach because they haven't learned that sexuality is still a taboo subject in our society. They accept the information very matter-of-factly and are incredibly open to learning about their bodies. For example, when I tell a group of kids in Kindergarten or Grade 1 (aged 5 or 6) that I'm going to teach them how to be body scientists, that I'm going to teach them scientific information about the body and scientific words for body parts, they love the idea. They hang on to my every word as if it's the most interesting thing they've ever heard!

In a Grade 1 class recently, as we were talking about how reproduction between a man and woman usually happens through sexual intercourse, one of the girls asked, "What if a lady has two men in her vagina? Will they both deliver sperm?" I explained that only one man's penis can be in a woman's vagina and deliver sperm at a time. She then continued, "But what if one man delivers the sperm and then another one does right after?" Before I could respond, another student interrupted and very calmly reasoned, "Well, I guess the baby gets two dads!" The other students nodded their heads in agreement.

In another class, after complimenting a Grade 1 student on how much body science information he already knew, he replied, "Thanks! It's my hobby. I love to gather information about the human body!"

By the time kids get to Grade 4 or 5 (age 9 and 10), however, it's a different story. These students are totally disgusted by anything to do with bodies, and S-E-X puts them right over the edge. They can be extremely embarrassed, and sometimes this discomfort manifests as lots of giggling and silliness. Parents tell me all the time that their preteens just don't want to talk to them about sexual health, and that they are at a loss when it comes to how to start the conversation.

This is when we, as parents and educators, need to get a little creative in terms of how we talk to kids. Rather than reading a body science book with our primaries before they go to bed, now we may have to get the books from the library or bookstore and leave them around the house for our intermediates to read. Of course, it's never too late to teach our kids about healthy sexuality, but normalizing the topic of sexual health at an early age in our homes makes the job of teaching so much easier through the tougher years of their development.

> I think that this is the great chance for us to learning this kind of staff so maybe in the future that you can take care of yourself carefully.

> How can I talk to my mom about this kind of stuff?

> Thank you for coming and teaching me important topics about me and the future.

And the good news is that you can't tell a child too much; they'll absorb whatever they're ready for at the time, and everything else will just go right over their heads. One time in a Grade 2 class (age 7), after spending about 20 minutes talking about bodies with a penis and testicles versus bodies with a uterus, vagina and ovaries using pictures in my pop-up book, one of the girls raised her hand and very skeptically asked, "If babies are born with no hair, how would the doctor know if it's a boy or a girl?" Clearly, the genital discussion went right over her head, but maybe she'll get it next time. At the very least, just by talking openly about her body we have sent her the positive message that bodies aren't a secret and that she has a right to learn about her body and how it works and how to take care of it, just like she would learn about anything else in science. Now *that's* powerful!

We also know from research done all over the world that talking about healthy bodies and healthy sexuality with young children does *not* in any way lead to early sexual experimentation and activity – in fact, the opposite is true. A World Health Organization literature review concluded that there is "no support for the contention that sex education encourages experimentation or increased activity. If any effect is observed, almost without exception, it is in the direction of postponed initiation of sexual intercourse and/or effective use of contraceptives." Teens and young adults who have learned in an open way at home are far less sexually active and unsafe in relationships. They also feel more secure, happy, and successful in their daily lives.

In a 2012 survey by the National Campaign to End Teen and Unplanned Pregnancy in the U.S., 87% of teenagers said "open, honest" conversations with their parents could help them put off sex and avoid pregnancy. We also know from the National Survey of Family Growth in the U.S. that students who take part in comprehensive sexual health education programs delay having sex for the first time, have less sex and fewer partners, and use contraception more consistently (and therefore experience fewer pregnancies) than their peers. Not surprisingly, abstinence-only education has not succeeded in delaying sexual activity and may even cause harm. It's been proven to be an epic fail.

It's not knowledge and information but *lack* of it (as well as curiosity) that leads to early exploration. Kids who learn about sexual health at a young age from reliable adults in their lives don't feel the need to experiment, because they know where to go (and *who to go to*) to get their questions answered. On the other hand, uninformed children are the ones who are more driven to Google "boobies" at a playdate; or to watch online pornography in Grade 8; or to experiment not only sexually at parties, but with other risk-taking behaviours because they feel that's what they need to do to get the information they want and need.

■ PARENTS VS. THE PLAYGROUND

The second reason we need to teach our children about healthy bodies and healthy sexuality at a young age is because if *we* don't teach them, somebody else will do it for us. Kids need years to understand and absorb the information we give them, including our family values and beliefs. We can't let an informant on the playground, on the Internet, or in the media get to them first with myths, misunderstandings, and exploitation. And I think we all agree that the world is a much different place than when we were growing up.

I often think about what my parents had to contend with when I was a preteen. Did they ever have it easy! Take TV, for example. I think the raciest shows we ever saw were *Love Boat* and *Fantasy Island* on a Saturday night. And I never even got to watch *Fantasy Island* because it was on at 10 p.m., which was way too late (obviously long before the age of PVRs and Netflix). Today our kids can access pretty much anything on TV at any time, even with parental control mechanisms in place. And I think some of the shows on the Family Channel are questionable in terms of their humour and adult storylines, not to mention the most sexually immature shows, such as *Family Guy* and *Two and a Half Men*. I can't tell you how many questions I get from students as a direct result of watching those shows, not to mention the nature and lyrics of songs on the radio. But I'll save that for another chapter.

We also have to remember that kids are exposed to much more than we think, sooner than we think. A few years ago, I was teaching a group of kindergarten kids and, as we were discussing the baby growing in the uterus, a girl exclaimed quite matter-of-factly, "And you know what else, Saleema? Sometimes grown-ups have sex when they're drunk."

I also remember a few years ago when my youngest stepdaughter, Kate, was 11. We were on spring break at a restaurant looking at the menu and, seemingly out of the blue, she asked, "What's S&M?" My husband nearly fell off his chair as I (relatively) calmly asked where she had heard that term. Pretty quickly it dawned on me that Rihanna's song on the radio at that time had the same title. No wonder she was asking!

Obviously, as parents, we need to create boundaries in terms of what our kids are exposed to on TV or anywhere else, especially when they're young. But children don't live in a bubble, and even if parents don't allow TV or much access to the Internet, children hear about all of this on the playground. And, trust me, they have lots of questions, even if they aren't asking. We always need to stay one step ahead of the game with accurate information, so that our kids know where to go with their questions, and so that they can also begin to think critically about what they see and hear. We need to teach them early on that we want them to come to us.

But some kids won't ask questions. They just aren't curious about their bodies because sexual health isn't on their radar. Some kids have already had their questions answered on the Internet or by an informant on the playground. Others get the message from parents, even if it's unintentional, that, for whatever reason, they don't want to talk or the kids shouldn't ask questions. Silence becomes a profound message to the child that the topic is off limits. "My family doesn't talk about this; it must be bad, and I'll be in big trouble if I mention it, or ask about it."

Once in a while I meet parents who say, "I want to be the first to tell my child about the facts of life." Great! If you want to be the first, then talk sex *today*! Grab the next opportunity, start talking, and don't be afraid to teach family values and beliefs, too. Kids need guidelines and they appreciate reasonable limits.

If children are asking questions without prompting, this is a great chance for parents to give information. It is also a huge compliment, because if our kids ask us questions it means they trust us as a credible source of information. Even more important than what we say when we're answering questions, though, is that we're *honest*. I remember a few years when ago a friend called me in panic one morning. On their way to school as they were listening to the radio, her nine-year-old daughter asked, "Mom, what's a 'ho'?" Knowing that her daughter was referring to a short form of the word "whore" but not wanting to get into it in the chaos of the carpool, my friend calmly replied, "Well, a hoe is a gardening tool." Now she was asking me if she "did good." My concern, of course, was that her daughter would find out, probably by recess, what a "ho" really is. After that, would the daughter come to her mom with her next question? Not if she can't count on mom to tell the truth.

When I'm working with parents, I assure them that they shouldn't expect to be able to answer questions with perfect eloquence right on the spot. If a tough one comes up and you have no idea how to respond, it is perfectly okay to say, **"I'm so glad you asked me that question, and I know you deserve a scientific answer. Let me think about how best to answer it for you. We'll talk about it (insert appropriate time…before bed, while we walk the dog, when our guests leave…).** It's better to take a step back and think about what you want to say than try to answer on the spot when you are flustered and taken off guard.

Of course, we don't want to send the message to our kids that this is a topic people should feel nervous or uncomfortable talking about. And if you answer a question and, reflecting back, you think you did a lousy job, it's never too late to fix it. You can always go back to your child and say, **"Remember this morning when I answered your question about a 'ho'? I'd like to try again."** Chances are your child has already moved on, but you'll feel better!

Parents also tell me that their kids appreciate their honesty when they say, **"I didn't get this body science when I was your age, so it's a bit tough for me to know how to teach you. But I recognize how important it is for you to learn this information and I'm going to do the very best I can."**

And don't forget your sense of humour when answering even the toughest questions. Bedtime is a great time to talk to littles, because they'll do anything to stop you from leaving and turning out the light. This is a good time to get a book and read with them, or to answer questions they may have asked earlier that day on a crowded bus or at Christmas dinner.

That reminds me, when talking about sex with kids at every stage of development, it's important to teach good manners and privacy.

For example, you could say, "I'm so glad we're having this conversation, because I want you to be safe and protected. But it wouldn't be a good idea to go to school tomorrow and tell your friends what we talked about because maybe they're not body scientists yet. We'll wait for adults in their lives to have a chance to teach them."

At the end of all my sessions with kids, I say something like, "**As body scientists, we have to be good judges of when it is appropriate to talk about bodies, and when is not. On the playground at recess, or at soccer practice, at a birthday party, or on the bus wouldn't be appropriate. Not that anything about bodies is a secret; it's just a private topic. Plus, when kids and teenagers talk about bodies without adults around, information gets really confusing and sometimes even scary. Your body is too important to be confused or scared about.**"

We also should stress the importance of going to a reliable adult with questions. A parent could say, "I'm so impressed that you're mature enough to ask such great scientific questions, and I hope you feel comfortable coming to me anytime there's something you want to know. But would it be a good idea to Google questions about your body? No, because we know that much of the 'information' we find online isn't true. Or would I want you to ask your older brother questions about your body? No, because although he means well, teenagers get confused sometimes. I think you deserve to know the truth, so always come to me (or your teacher, or your doctor, or another reliable adult) when you have questions."

In perfect world, one that's truly sexually mature, any adult could answer a child's questions with science and health information. But there are incorrect assumptions out there; for example, dads should talk to their sons and moms should talk to their daughters. The best scenario would be one where every parent feels comfortable talking to their children, and in families with two parents, it would be a team effort. And don't forget that other trusted, reliable adults in your child's life are invaluable, not only when it comes to answering questions, but reinforcing the information you've given them.

■ KNOWLEDGE IS PROTECTION

The third reason we need to start from day one to teach our children about healthy bodies and healthy sexuality is that studies from all over the world consistently show that kids who learn scientific words for body parts, and that they own their bodies, are better protected from sexual abuse. Children need this information to help them avoid exploitative situations, especially when we aren't around.

Meg Hickling tells us that she often used to visit prisons. She hated going, but she went whenever she was invited because the inmates taught her so much about how they trick, trap, and seduce children into abuse. Offenders become very skillful at choosing vulnerable children – most have been abused themselves so they know exactly what to look for. What they know is that children who are sexually aware and have scientific vocabulary for body parts have been taught by parents or other reliable adults in their lives. They have probably also been instructed to report to someone else should something exploitative happen. A child who doesn't know anything probably also hasn't been taught to report and, therefore, is an easy target for abuse.

A story a parent told me years ago is a sad example of this. She worked at a daycare and one morning a four-year-old boy told one of the other workers, "My grandpa was playing with my toy last night." She replied, "Oh that's nice," and went on with her busy day. But within a three-week period, that boy told every one of the workers there the same thing. Finally, they called his parents in to find that, in their family, the penis was referred to as "the toy." How tragic that this four-year-old boy was brave enough to disclose the abuse, but wasn't armed with the vocabulary to let the adults in his life know what was happening.

Providing sexual health and safety information is especially important for children with physical and developmental differences, as research indicates that they experience up to five times more abuse than other children. These kids are also at greater risk as teens and adults, because they're often taught to be passive and obedient, and to trust all caregivers. They may also lack boundaries and communication skills that help keep them safe. It's crucial to remember that children with special needs are sexual beings, just like everybody else. They usually go through puberty at exactly the same time as other children do, and they have similar questions about growing up. Positive messages about sexual health and safety need to be given again and again, with patience, humour, and compassion.

■ THE STAGES OF SEXUAL DEVELOPMENT: WHAT TO TEACH AND WHEN

Now that we understand how important it is to start teaching our kids about sexual health at an early age, the next logical question is, "*What* do we teach, and *when*?" Of course, children don't mature overnight and so their education doesn't have to happen all at once. We can pace ourselves, building on the information and skills we teach them as they get older. Based on research from all over the world on the sexual development of children, as well as her extensive experience teaching children of all ages, Meg Hickling developed five stages of sexual development that children grow through as they come to understand sexuality in a mature way. We see these stages as pads in a lily pond. Everyone spends time on the various pads at different points depending on the situation, and our own education, experience, and maturity.

Imagine a lily pond with "nirvana," the sexually-mature-adult island, in the middle. The ideal situation would be to spend as much time there as possible. Closest to the shore are the preschooler pads. Into the pond a bit, but not far, are the primary pads. In the middle are the intermediate pads. And closest to the sexually-mature-adult island are the adolescent pads. Sometimes, through lack of education or life experience, people get stuck on one pad for a long time, or forever. Some people continually hop back and forth, never coming close to or reaching sexual maturity. And some are kept, by circumstances they can't control, on one or two pads.

In the following chapters, I'll be writing about the stages of sexual development that children and teens go through in most countries today. But in countries such as Sweden, Holland, and Germany, where sexual health education has been mandatory in schools for several generations, children don't go through the magical thinking of the preschoolers, the bathroom humour of the primaries, or the "gross-me-outs" of the intermediates with anything like the intensity that children from other countries do. Today, most parents in Sweden, for example, were brought up by parents who were well informed and sexually mature themselves, who talked openly and factually about sexuality and sexual health, and who carried little of the emotional baggage, negativity, and shame that others have around the topic. The statistical evidence of health in this country is clear: lower rates of sexual abuse, sexual exploitation, abortion, suicide, teenage pregnancy, and STIs (sexually transmitted infections). Our goal here in Canada should be to learn by their example so that we can progress to new levels of sexual maturity.

2. Gender and Sexuality

2. Gender and Sexuality

■ CREATING A COMMON LANGUAGE

"What exactly does gender identity mean?"
"Is being transgender the same as being transsexual?"
"What the heck does cisgender mean?"
"How do we keep up with the latest acronyms used to refer to LGBTQ+ people?"

I hear these valid questions regularly from both parents and students, and I think it makes sense to address them before we get into the nitty-gritty of what to teach kids and when. That is, we need to be on the same page when it comes to what gender and sexuality mean. We also need to create a common language to use throughout this book: a language that promotes inclusivity, respect, and celebration of the complex, unique sexual beings we are at every stage of life. Anna Soole, one of our gifted iGirl educators, has taught me an immeasurable amount about inclusive language and has been a huge support in writing this chapter.

I've chosen "The Genderbread Person (v 3.3)" graphic to use as a framework for our discussion of gender and sexuality. This version of The Genderbread Person was created by Sam Killermann, a social justice comedian who talks about gender, sexuality, identity, and privilege both in his shows and on his website, www.itspronounced metrosexual.com.

Before we dive in, I want to mention that the Genderbread Person has faced some valid criticism over the years. Some people have noted that Killermann doesn't give credit to those who were

The Genderbread Person v3.3

by it's pronounced METROsexual.com

Gender is one of those things everyone thinks they understand, but most people don't. Like inception. Gender isn't binary. It's not either/or. In many cases it's both/and. A bit of this, a dash of that. This tasty little guide is meant to be an appetizer for gender understanding. It's okay if you're hungry for more. In fact, that's the idea.

- - - Identity
- - - Attraction
- - - Expression
- - - Sex

Gender Identity
⊘ → Woman-ness
⊘ → Man-ness

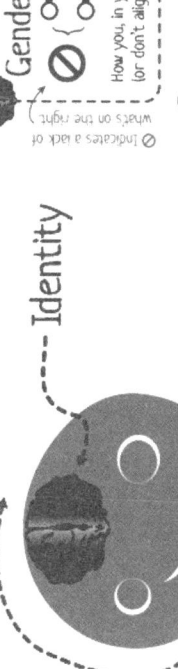

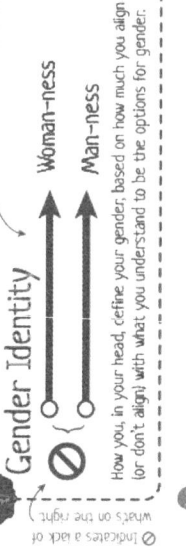

How you, in your head, define your gender, based on how much you align (or don't align) with what you understand to be the options for gender.

Gender Expression
⊘ → Feminine
⊘ → Masculine

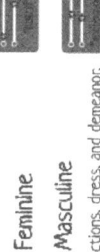

The ways you present gender, through your actions, dress, and demeanor, and how those presentations are interpreted based on gender norms.

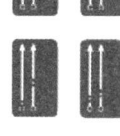

Biological Sex
⊘ → Female-ness
⊘ → Male-ness

The physical sex characteristics you're born with and develop, including genitalia, body shape, voice pitch, body hair, hormones, chromosomes, etc.

Plot a point on both continua in each category to represent your identity, combine all ingredients to form your Genderbread.

4 (of infinite) possible plot and label combos

⊘ Indicates a lack of what's on the right.

Romantically Attracted to
Nobody → (Women/Females/Femininity)
Nobody → (Men/Males/Masculinity)

Sexually Attracted to
Nobody → (Women/Females/Femininity)
Nobody → (Men/Males/Masculinity)

In each grouping, circle all that apply to you and plot a point, depicting the aspects of gender toward which you experience attraction.

For a bigger bite, read more at http://bit.ly/genderbread

instrumental in creating the original version of the framework (a southern California social working group as early as 2005, and several gender and sexuality minority community members since then). Others feel that such a framework excludes too many people's experience of gender and sexuality because there will never be clearly delineated categories into which all people will fit. This is important to acknowledge and consider when using the Genderbread Person as a tool for understanding.

I've chosen to use Killermann's version because it's the most comprehensive tool I've seen, insightful, and easy to understand, especially for people who have not thought much about gender and sexuality. It's not perfect, but it works well as an introduction to some complex ideas.

Let's break this down into bite-sized pieces, one section at a time. Please keep in mind that the four aspects of a person's sexuality that Sam outlines are *interrelated*, but not *interconnected*. What he means is that gender identity, gender expression, biological sex, and sexual attraction are independent of one another, and therefore they don't determine one another. For example, just because someone identifies as a female doesn't mean that they always wear traditionally feminine clothes or are always sexually attracted to males. Someone who identifies as a straight male may have a more feminine demeanor or style of dressing.

Gender identity refers to how you feel about yourself in terms of being a man or a woman, both, or something different entirely. More and more, we recognize that not all people fit the *gender binary* of "man" or "woman", and may feel that they're somewhere in between, or are something else entirely. For example, they may identify as *genderqueer*. *Two-spirit* is a sacred term used only by Indigenous people to describe themselves, among other things, as genderqueer. It's also important to note that some people don't feel as if they are on the man-woman continuum at all and may identify as *agender, third-gender,* or *bigender* among other terms. I like the idea that our range of gender identities can be expressed as a kaleidoscope, with countless possibilities in a 3-D spectrum.

33

TALK
SEX
TODAY

FUN FACT:
We know now that gender identity is formed by the age of three and is very difficult to change. We also know that the formation of gender identity is affected by hormones and environment just as much as it is by biology. This is all fine, except when someone is assigned a gender at birth based on their physical body, but that isn't consistent with how they identify in the future. More on that in a bit.

34

TALK SEX TODAY

***Gender expression* refers to how you act, dress, behave, and interact to demonstrate your gender.** It can be intentional or unintentional, and is interpreted by others based on traditional gender roles (i.e., men wear pants, women wear dresses). Gender expression is fluid in that it can be more masculine or more feminine from day to day and even from outfit to outfit. For example, you could wear sweat pants and a T-shirt (traditionally masculine) during the day and then put on a dress (traditionally feminine) to go out for dinner.

Someone who expresses themselves equally as masculine and feminine may call themselves *androgenous*. Someone who expresses their gender neither as masculine nor feminine may call themselves *gender neutral*. It's interesting (and sad and frustrating) to note that in

> *Is it possible for a women to give birth to a child that is a girl on the inside and a boy on the outside? If yes why?*

our culture it's much more acceptable for a female to express her gender in a more masculine way than is typical for females than it is for a male to express his gender in a more feminine way. That is, a girl who would rather play "Capture the Flag" in the muddy playing field at recess than play with My Little Ponies is referred to as a tomboy – a cute, empowering term for "a girl who does boy stuff." The only term there is for "a boy who does girl stuff" is fag – a derogatory term (in this context, anyway) also used to denote weakness. While it's perfectly acceptable (and even celebrated) for girls to want to be a Mutant Ninja Turtle for Halloween, a boy who wants to dress up like Strawberry Shortcake certainly wouldn't get the same response (though this is changing a bit).

The reason for this difference, at least in part, is due to the power of *gender stereotypes* in our society. Gender stereotypes are strict rules that society teaches us, from the day we are born, about how to dress, think, and act in order to be a "real girl" or a "real boy." Gender stereotypes teach us that any departure from these rules is unacceptable, which is why so many people, even today, don't feel safe expressing their true gender identity. I'll say more in a later chapter about how gender stereotypes can be damaging at all ages and why we need to challenge them.

Biological sex* refers to your biology or anatomy (organs, hormones, and chromosomes). According to Killermann, being female means having a vagina, uterus, ovaries, two X chromosomes, and predominant estrogen. Being male, on the other hand, means having testicles, a penis, an XY chromosome configuration, and predominant testosterone. Simple, right? Not so much.

Sexual organs may not be strictly male or female. For example, among many possibilities, someone can look like a male at birth (with a penis and testicles) but have a functional female reproductive system inside their body. And others have genital characteristics that may resemble both males and females in some way. We call this *intersex*.

You may have heard the term hermaphrodite used to describe a person who is intersex. Unfortunately, this word has been used to stigmatize and harm intersex people, and so it is no longer an appropriate term to use. Slang terms like *he/she* and *ladyman*, used to refer to people who are intersex, are also disrespectful and inappropriate.

Still with me? Good, because here's where things get even more beautifully complex. Remember earlier when I mentioned that someone can be assigned a gender at birth, based on their physical body, which doesn't jive with their gender identity as they grow up? For example, they may feel like a girl but be perceived by others as a boy, or vice versa. These people often identify as *transgender* or *trans*. If they choose, people who are transgender can transition from being male to female, or female to male. This process may or may not involve treatments, medication, and surgery to change their body physically. A transgender person who has altered their body physically as part of this transition may (or may not) call themselves *transsexual*.

* Some people are uncomfortable using the term "biological sex" to refer to one's physical body. They argue that sex is partly biological, but also culturally constructed and, therefore, not "objectively measurable." So the term is viewed by some to represent only a part of the full picture.

Because we know that gender identity, gender expression, and one's physical body at birth are not always in sync, we can't assume, for example, that *all* girls get periods and that *all* boys get wet dreams. Nor can we assume that *all* women have a uterus and ovaries, and that *all* men have a penis and testicles. The truth is, people who are born with a uterus and ovaries *usually* get periods and are *usually* assigned female at birth. People who are born with a penis and testicles *usually* get wet dreams and are *usually* assigned male at birth. Doctors and parents may still assign people who are born with ambiguous genitals a gender that they may or may not identify with later. This can be damaging and traumatizing, especially if the assignment at birth includes surgery.

> Wouldn't it be easier if your gender wasn't based on your genitals?

Out of respect and with the intent of including people who are transgender and intersex, we need to reflect this scientific fact in our everyday language, and in what we teach our children about sexual health. Although attitudes are slowly changing, transgender people have endured discrimination, harassment, and inequality for years. Thankfully, though, as with many other human rights issues, we're making progress; more and more people understand the importance of honouring how every person identifies sexually. But (even for me as an educator), knowing what is appropriate language to use when referring to or communicating with transgender people can be tricky. I continue to learn from transgender people and their experience. Here's what they tell me they appreciate.

Avoid using the phrase "sex change." Instead, say "transition."

Avoid using the terms "transgendered" or "transgenderism." Instead, say "a transgender person" or "a person who is transgender."

Avoid using the terms "biologically male," "biologically female," "born a man," and "born a woman." Instead, say "assigned male at birth," "assigned female at birth," "designated male at birth," or "designated female at birth."

Always use a transgender person's chosen name. Even if they haven't obtained a legal name change, call them what they wish to be called.

Whenever possible, ask transgender people which pronoun they would like you to use. If it isn't appropriate to ask, use the pronoun that is consistent with the person's appearance and gender expression. And use "they/their" instead of "he/his" or "she/her."

Let's talk about the term *cisgender*. When someone's gender identity is consistent with the gender they were assigned at birth, they are cisgender. For example, I am cisgender. My physical body is consistent with being female and the gender I identify with is female too.

The cisgender identity comes with a lot of privileges, many of which we cisgender people take for granted or simply don't notice. Consider these, for example. A cisgender person can

- use clearly marked public restrooms without confusion, fear of verbal abuse, or physical intimidation
- feel valid as a man or woman regardless of how much surgery they've had or how much they do or don't look cisgender
- walk through the mall without being stared at or whispered about because of how they look
- reasonably assume that they won't miss out on a job opportunity or a mortgage on the basis of their gender identity and expression
- buy clothes and shoes that fit off the rack without salespeople questioning their choices
- be spared having to explain their "situation" at family gatherings
- be referred to using their chosen pronouns without having to offer an explanation
- enjoy the simplicity of their anatomy and gender being consistent when talking to children about bodies without feeling the need to address the complexities of the issue

We need to be more mindful of these things if we're going to make the world a more transgender-friendly place.

***Sexual attraction* (or *sexual orientation* as it's often called) refers to who you are sexually (physically) attracted to.** This is different than *romantic attraction,* which refers to emotional and spiritual attraction to women/females/femininity or men/males/masculinity. We need to remember, though, that some people aren't romantically attracted to any of these characteristics. Also, some people are romantically attracted to something else entirely.

We need to consider both sexual attraction and romantic attraction. We used to think, for example, that if you're male and you're romantically and sexually attracted only to females, you're *straight or heterosexual.* If you're a person who is romantically or sexually attracted to both males and females, you're *bisexual* (often known as "bi"). And if you're a male who is attracted only to males, you're *gay or homosexual* (*lesbian* is a term used to refer specifically to a gay female).

More and more, however, we're understanding that it's not that cut and dried. In fact, thanks to groundbreaking research by Dr. Alfred Kinsey in the 1940s and 1950s, and the experiential testimonies of countless queer and trans people, we now know that people don't necessarily fit neatly into one of the above three categories. That is, each of us exists at our own unique place in the kaleidoscope of romantic and sexual attraction.

We also know that someone can be romantically attracted to one sex, but sexually attracted to another. For example, a person may identify as a man who has sex with men (MSM). They want to be in a relationship with a woman because of romantic feelings, but are also (or exclusively) sexually attracted to other men.

As well, it's important to recognize that about 1% of people report feeling no sexual attraction at all to others. They are *asexual.* Many asexual people feel romantic attraction to others and identify as gay, straight, bi, panromantic, queer, or something different entirely. They enjoy all of the romantic aspects of a healthy relationship, but don't have sexual feelings and aren't into sex. This isn't the same as being *celibate,* which refers to a conscious choice not to have sex despite having sexual feelings. Asexual people may masturbate, but cite doing so for relaxation, not sexual release. Interestingly, we also know from research that asexual people respond physiologically to sexual arousal and are able to have sex, orgasm, and reproduce (and many of them do).

Though they don't find their lack of sexual attraction problematic, asexual people often face discrimination from those around them. Although disproven in research, critics claim that people are asexual as a result of childhood abuse, that asexuality is related to anxiety or depression, is a severe sexual dysfunction that needs to be cured, or that it doesn't exist at all. In response, a large online community called AVEN (Asexual Visibility and Education Network) offers support with the goal of increasing visibility and inclusion of asexual people.

Before we move on, we need to tackle those LGBTQ+ acronyms. I don't blame parents who feel overwhelmed trying to figure out which one to use; even I have a hard time keeping up with the changes. But here's what I know. These acronyms are an important and valuable attempt to create an exhaustive representation of all identities, expressions, and attractions in the kaleidoscope of gender and sexuality. The relatively recent addition of the "+" at the end is meant to include possibilities beyond being Lesbian, Gay, Bisexual, Transgender, or Queer.

Inclusivity superstars would use the acronym LGBPTTQQIIAA+. These letters stand for lesbian, gay, bisexual, pansexual, transgender, transsexual, queer, questioning, intersex, intergender, asexual, and ally.

I've discussed most of these terms throughout this chapter, but just to fill in the blanks, *pansexual* refers to someone who experiences sexual, romantic, physical, and/or spiritual attraction toward members of all gender identities and expressions. Although the term *queer* used to be a derogatory slang term used to identify LGBTQ+ people, it's been reclaimed by the LGBTQ+ community as a symbol of pride, representing all individuals who don't identify with gender and sexuality "norms." A person who is *questioning* is in the process of exploring their sexual attraction or gender identity. *Intergender* people have a gender identity that falls somewhere between the binary genders of female and male. And an *ally* is a straight person who supports queer people. (That's what I strive to be!)

I mention this acronym not because I expect anyone to memorize it (chances are it will have changed by the time this book goes to print anyway). More important than the specific acronym we use is that we talk and act in the spirit of inclusion, and that we celebrate diversity. And if you're ever stuck, just use LGBTQ+.

Finally, I want to mention two more terms: *cross-dresser* or *transvestite*. Historically, these terms have been used to refer to someone who wears clothes designed for the opposite sex. Today they are felt by some people to be offensive. So let's not use them anymore.

I know that's a pretty intense way to start what I promise will be an easy-to-read, lighthearted book. And this wasn't even an exhaustive list of all the awesome, inclusive terms you may come across. But this stuff is so important that it deserves to go first. Plus, now we have a common language, a context that we can use to look at gender and sexuality as inclusively and respectfully as possible. Love it!

■ RESOURCES

FOR PARENTS

WEBSITES
- www.itspronouncedmetrosexual.com
- www.pflagcanada.ca
- www.genderspectrum.org
- www.belongto.org
- www.bcchildrens.ca
- www.transstudent.org
- www.imatyfa.org
- www.glaad.com
- www.asexuality.com
- www.genderqueerid.com

BOOKS
- *Supporting Transgender and Gender Creative Youth: Schools, Families and Communities in Action*, by Elizabeth J. Meyer and Annie Pullen Sansfacon.

FOR CHILDREN

BOOKS
- *Sex Is a Funny Word: A Book about Bodies, Feelings, and You*, by Cory Silverberg. An awesome, trans-inclusive body book for kids.

BOOKS THAT ARE RACIALLY DIVERSE AND LGBTQ+ POSITIVE, FROM PUBLISHER FLAMINGO RAMPANT
- *A Princess of Great Daring*, by Tobi Hill-Meyer. This is about a young trans girl, Jamie, and her three best friends who are playing princes, knights, and princesses. But it's not your average "rescue the princess" story.

- *Is That for a Boy or a Girl?* by S. Bear Bergman. This is a book of short poems about gender-independent kids and what they like to do or wear. Spoiler alert: there *aren't* "boy things" and "girl things."
- *Love Is in the Hair*, by Sryus Ware. This is about a little girl waiting for her sibling to be born whose gay uncles tell her stories about their family through objects woven into their dreadlocks.
- *M Is for Mustache,* by Catherine Hernandez. This is an ABC book about a girl and her chosen family and how they celebrate Pride.
- *Zero Dads Club*, by Angel Adehoya. This is about a group of kids who self-organize and do a special project while their class makes Father's Day cards.

BOOKS THAT CELEBRATE DIVERSE FAMILIES
- *Asha's Mums*, by Rosamund Elwin.
- *How Would You Feel If Your Dad Was Gay?* by Ann Heron.
- *Making Love Visible: In Celebration of Gay and Lesbian Families*, by Jean Swallow.
- *Molly's Family*, by Nancy Garden.
- *The Different Dragon*, by Jennifer Bryan.
- *What Makes a Baby?* by Cory Silverberg.
- *While You Were Sleeping*, by Stephanie Burks.

FOR TEENS

BOOKS
- *Beautiful Music for Ugly Children*, by Kirstin Cronn-Mills.
- *Beyond Magenta: Transgender Teens Speak Out*, by Susan Kuklin.

3. The Magical Thinkers

3. The Magical Thinkers

■ PRESCHOOLERS (PRESCHOOL–GRADE 1)

You may be wondering why we include K–Grade 1 students in the preschool stage of development. Although I strongly encourage parents to start teaching basic body science to children as young as age two, we also teach these concepts to kindergarten and Grade 1 children in the classroom. These kids are magical thinkers, too, and "preschool" information serves as a good foundation to build upon as they move through elementary school.

■ MAGICAL THINKING 101

When preschoolers don't have factual information, they make up a story to explain things to themselves. Educational psychologists call this *magical thinking*. Preschoolers do a lot of magical thinking around reproduction if no one tells them the truth. Some decide that if you want a baby you go to the hospital. The hospital, they imagine, has rooms full of babies and the nurses hand them out to anyone who asks for one.

One mother courageously confessed to Meg that she'd found herself stuck at this stage. She told her son that she was going to the hospital to get a baby and he said he'd like a boy baby, not a girl baby. She said, "I'll see what I can do." When she brought home a baby girl, he said, "I don't want a baby sister; take it back and change it." She told him that the hospital was all out of boy babies and they had to take this one. Stork stories and cabbage patches are all examples of adults doing magical thinking because they aren't comfortable and mature enough themselves to tell the truth.

But when adults are honest and say, **"When a man and a woman want to make a baby, what usually happens is they put the penis inside the vagina to deliver the sperm to the egg,"** preschoolers look at them like they're talking about bicycle safety. There's no silliness, and no giggling; it's just science to them. And very quickly, they're ready to move on. One time, after explaining how babies are made to a group of preschoolers, I asked if anyone had any questions. One of the boys raised his hand and said, "Yah, I got a question. Can we do play centres now?"

The biggest challenge for adults when teaching kids this age is to be prepared to tell the story again and again. Preschoolers don't always understand the information fully the first time, or they only take in a bit of what was said, or more commonly, some other person comes along with a better story and they choose to believe it instead.

But preschoolers are the easiest of all children to teach about sexual health. As I mentioned earlier, they carry no emotional baggage around sexuality and they haven't learned yet that it's still a taboo subject in our society.

The best thing about this age is that preschoolers have so much intellectual curiosity – they want to know exactly how it all works. A few years ago, I was teaching some preschoolers and I had just explained how babies are usually made. Before I could continue, one of the girls interrupted me and wanted to clarify, "So the man puts his penis into the vagina?" I replied, "Yes, sometimes." Looking perplexed, she responded, "Well then how would he get it back on?" I simply explained that the penis isn't detachable and she seemed fine with that. Preschoolers accept information about their bodies in the same matter-of-fact way they accept information about anything else, so why not share it?

> *Why do moms and dads lie about where babys come from*

SAFETY FIRST: ABUSE PREVENTION

The first thing I share with students of all ages is the fact that there are three private parts on the human body – the mouth, the breasts, and the genitals (everything between a person's legs, from the belly button, through the legs and up to the lower back). I explain that these parts of the body are private because no one can go in them or on them without permission. Sometimes parents ask me why I say "go on" rather than "touch." The reason is that abuse isn't limited to touching. It could involve putting a body part in someone's mouth, or placing a whole body on another's body. Equally important is to stress that our bodies are never a secret from ourselves; we can look at and touch our bodies whenever we want to, as long as we're in private. Our bodies belong to us and sometimes it feels good to explore them.

When I ask preschoolers how they would react should someone go on their body in a way that they know is inappropriate or that feels uncomfortable, they tell me they would yell and scream and go tell a parent. And they're exactly right. I let them know that they're allowed to do anything they can to get away from a person who is doing this. I instruct them to tell the person "No!" or "Stop!" in a really bossy voice. And it doesn't matter who this person is. Even if it's someone they know, like a family friend or a relative, they're allowed to do anything they can to get away from that person. If the person doesn't listen to their words, they need to use their body to get away. Of course, using violence isn't usually the way we solve problems, but if this is the only way they can get to safety, then it's allowed.

Once they get away, I tell children to immediately report the incident to an adult they trust. Even if the person has threatened them to keep it a secret, they need to report what happened. The reason for this is that it's not a problem that kids, or even teenagers, can deal with alone. Plus, there are no secrets when it comes to people going on kids' private parts. We want them to tell us so that we can make sure they get the help and support they need to deal with their experience. I stress that they should never get in trouble for this; they haven't done anything wrong. This message is especially important because most abusers are known to the victim. When this is the case, reporting is more difficult because the child might be afraid of being blamed, or causing problems in a family, or that someone they know and like may get in big trouble.

I also tell children that if the person they report to doesn't take them seriously, or doesn't do anything to help them right away, they need to keep telling and telling until someone *does* listen to them and *does* do something. Of course, we don't want to scare our children unnecessarily, so we can put it in perspective by comparing having this information to doing a fire drill, or earthquake drill at school. It's all about safety.

■ CONSENT FOR PRESCHOOLERS

Even at this young age, we need to teach our children the basics of healthy consent. That is, when we give them permission to say "No!" to uncomfortable touching, we send the message that they're the boss of their bodies. No one is allowed to go on them without their consent. This can be tricky when, at bath time, a parent is trying to help their little one wash but they exclaim, "It's my body! You can't go on it without my permission!" You could simply respond to your smart little body scientist by saying, **"I'm so proud that you know that you are the boss of your body! As your parent, though, it's my job to help keep you clean. Would it be okay if I help you wash your genitals?"** If a child is extremely resistant, a parent could invite them to do it themselves with supervision. Of course, we should remind them why it's so important to keep all of our body parts (especially the genitals) clean.

Teaching consent to preschoolers extends beyond the bathtub to everyday interactions with others. For example, we can teach our kids the importance of asking before hugging or kissing their friends. Before leaving a play date, a child could say, "Can I hug you goodbye?" If the friend says "No," or shows discomfort, maybe they can offer a high five instead. Along the same lines, we should never force our children to hug or kiss anyone else. I vividly remember my parents' dinner parties when I was growing up. They were super fun and I loved the attention that was showered on me by my parents' friends. But at the end of the night, I was expected to walk around the room and give everyone a kiss and a hug goodbye. Some nights I felt fine doing this. Other nights, though, I didn't. But I wasn't allowed to change my mind; it wasn't my choice. Hugging and kissing was just the polite thing to do. Looking back, I would have appreciated some other options. And if friends or relatives are offended by a lack of physical affection from a child, you can explain what you're doing. If they don't understand, well, quite frankly, that's their problem.

The basic concept "No Means No" should also apply to interactive play between young children. Parents can explain that if a friend says "No," we need to stop what we are doing immediately. Similarly, if we say "No," our friend needs to listen. If they don't stop when we ask, we need to consider whether we feel safe playing with them. Parents may need to intervene if the message needs to be reinforced. "No" is an important safe word. This also shows support for the child and is a good way to model assertiveness.

Also doable, even at this age, is to teach our children to interpret non-verbal cues. Just because someone doesn't say "No," or "Stop," doesn't mean they feel good about what's happening. Recognizing emotions like discomfort, uncertainty, anxiety, sadness, and anger in others through facial expressions and other non-verbal communication is a helpful skill to have at any age. And if our child knows that their friend is struggling, encourage empathy and offer ways to help them.

Teaching our children to recognize and trust their own emotions is equally important. Ask questions about how they're feeling, validate them, and support them in sorting their emotions out. Of course, sometimes emotions are confusing and difficult to describe or label; our gut is simply telling us that something isn't quite right. Those gut feelings also need to be trusted, especially if they're related to feeling uncomfortable or unsafe around certain people or situations. That is, if your child suddenly gets anxious when they're around a certain friend or relative, take it seriously and ask questions to get to the bottom of it.

■ THE ABCs OF GENDER STEREOTYPES

Gender stereotypes are the colour-coded boxes of rules we put people into, depending on whether they are assigned male or female at birth. Think about the clothes we typically buy for baby boys (blue) and baby girls (pink). Walk into a Lego store and you'll find a kit to build your own spaceship in the boys' section, and a kit to build your own hair salon in the girls' section. And movies and TV shows still feature the big strong man rescuing the helpless, weak, female victim. These gender stereotypes limit *all* of us. They prevent us from living as our true selves, ostracizing those who don't fit neatly or perfectly into the box they've been assigned to. Not to mention that those boxes don't honour the fact that some people don't identify as solely male or solely female. Even in preschool, children pick up on whether what they like and how they express themselves is "normal" for their gender.

Thankfully, more and more of us have started to challenge these limiting beliefs. Today, boys can wear pink and get away with it (most of the time). Most parents don't freak out (and instead embrace it) when their son wants to put nail polish on like his sister. Girls are being encouraged to participate in activities and pursue areas of study traditionally reserved for boys. Dads are taking paternity leave. Major department stores are reworking their toy sections to be gender neutral, and we've seen nationwide movements promoting the breaking down of gender stereotypes in schools and on social media (see examples at the end of this chapter). We're definitely on our way, but we still have work to do.

A 2011 Plan Canada report entitled "Because I Am a Girl: So What About Boys?" revealed that, compared to adults, youth have some very positive views on gender roles: 91% believe equality among men and women is good for everyone, and at least 96% of youth believe girls should have the same opportunities to make their own choices as boys. But the survey (of about 1,000 youth and 1,000 adults) shows stereotypes and inequalities still exist. One third of Canadian boys believe that a woman's most important role is to take care of the home; 48% of youth believe men should be the principal income earner; and at least 45% of Canadian kids believe men need to be tough. Yikes!

So what can we do? For starters, we as parents can be mindful of the messages we send to our kids about gender in how we live our day-to-day lives. Let's also ask questions about what our kids see when it comes to gender roles and representation:

- Do we treat our daughters differently than our sons?
- How are roles in our household divided? Do we assign chores differently for our daughters than our sons?
- As males, how do we treat our female partners, and vice versa?
- Do we steer our sons in the direction of certain toys and our daughters in another direction? And how are those toys marketed differently?
- Do we watch movies that perpetuate the notion of man as hero and woman as victim? Or do we balance those with movies featuring strong female characters (the few we can find, anyway!)?
- Do we allow our children to have choices around their interests and activities free from gender stereotypes?
- Would we be okay with our son wearing traditionally feminine clothes?
- How else are gender stereotypes (even unintentionally) reinforced in our home?

▪ HEAD AND SHOULDERS, KNEES AND ... TESTICLES?

In much the same way, all parents give messages to their kids about sexual health without even realizing it. Non-verbal messages through touching, day-to-day child-care, facial expressions, and actions say so much to little ones about sexual health. It would be helpful if parents could name the genitals as matter-of-factly as they name elbows. Think for a moment about how we teach babies to talk: "This is your nose; this is your chin; this is your belly button …" And then we make the giant leap to the knees. Or we use baby words like "dinky" and "pee-pee" and other slang names for private parts that have been passed down in the family for generations. One time, a Grade 1 boy bragged, "I know another word for my penis … 'my manhood'!" I wonder who taught him that? And one of the few things that I don't appreciate about Oprah is her excessive use of the slang "va-jay-jay" to refer to the vagina. She's made it trendy even for adults to use silly names for body parts. Not to mention, the correct word for what she's really referring to is "vulva"!

I don't want to be too hard on parents today, though, because, let's face it, most of us didn't grow up learning the technical terminology for body parts from our own parents. But we all need to learn the vocabulary and practice using it. When she was teaching, my good friend and colleague Alice Bell would urge parents to say penis 50 times in a row while vacuuming. Hopefully your neighbour won't stop by to borrow some sugar while you're doing it!

I hate to sound like a broken record, but this is about safety. Years ago, a woman approached me after a parent session at an elementary school. Sheepishly, she admitted that all these years she had been referring to her daughter's vagina as her "cookie jar." She understood now just how dangerous that was.

Start the day your baby is born by naming the genitals. "Let's wash your penis, let's wash your vulva (not vagina, which is an opening and unnecessary to wash)." Then by the time your child is old enough to ask, "Why do some people have a penis and some have a vulva?" you'll feel comfortable with the words. Now you just have to figure out how to put them all together!

As your child is able to understand more, you can give them more scientific information, such as, **"The penis is designed to deliver sperm to the egg in order to make a baby. It can deliver urine to the toilet, too, but you don't have to have a penis to urinate."**

■ BODIES WITH A PENIS AND TESTICLES

As we discussed in Chapter 2, how someone feels and expresses themselves as male, female, both, or something different entirely in relation to how their body looks physically is incredibly complex. For this reason, when talking about anatomy, it's inaccurate to say *all boys have this* and *all girls have that*. This is especially relevant for parents, given that children at increasingly young ages are open about being transgender or intersex. While they work for most people, for others the terms "boy" and "girl" are misleading, confusing, and exclusionary.

For readability, however, I'm going to use the terms "boy," "girl," "male," and "female," from time to time when talking about bodies. But please know that I'm using these terms to refer to one's physical body only. I recognize that a girl may never have a period if they were assigned male at birth. In the same way, a boy may never produce sperm if they were assigned female at birth. Every body is unique and beautiful and I celebrate these differences.

I tell children that the penis isn't just for decoration; it actually has the important purpose of delivering sperm. It can only do this when it's erect, so practice erections happen many times each day as a person is growing up. Daytime erections aren't as vigorous after puberty, but penises typically practice several erections during sleep.

TALK SEX TODAY

FUN FACT:
Penises begin to practice erections 17 weeks into pregnancy. Now that's planning ahead!

Penis

Urethra

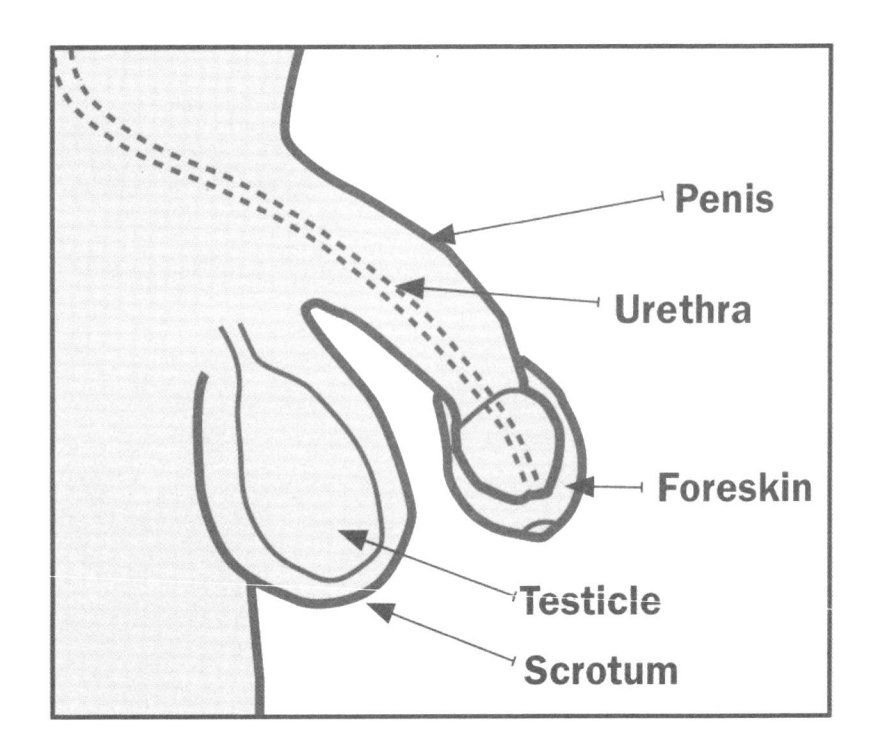

Foreskin

Testicle

Scrotum

A morning erection doesn't mean that your child has to go to the bathroom; they may have a full bladder when they wake up, but that's just a coincidence. When the penis gets erect, a valve at the mouth of the bladder closes tightly so that no urine can escape. It allows free passage of sperm through the urethra without contamination by urine. Nature wouldn't send a signal that you have to go to the bathroom and then turn off the waterworks!

Erections during childhood are often simply practice erections, and kids need to be reassured about them. If they aren't, the silence or an embarrassed reaction from others becomes a message of guilt, shame, and taboo. A couple years ago when I was in a Grade 1 class, one of the boys raised his hand and asked, "Saleema, why does my penis go hard sometimes?" His classmates nodded their heads, acknowledging his great scientific question, and I briefly explained that practice erections are a good sign that a penis is healthy, working properly, and may be preparing for making a baby some day. Immediately, the students started high-fiving the boy, celebrating the fact that their classmate's penis was healthy. As soon as they were finished, they went back to criss-cross applesauce (sitting legs crossed) on the carpet, eager to learn more body science.

Talk to your child about their penis – how it works, how to take care of it (wash it like a finger, the foreskin may not fully retract until after puberty), and help them to feel comfortable so that if they get an infection or injury they'll be able to tell you right away without embarrassment.

It's also a good idea to explain circumcision. Young children see both circumcised and uncircumcised penises (although rates of circumcision have dramatically decreased in Canada over the last decade), often when they're in a changing room after swimming or playing sports. Here's what I say to children who have questions:

"There's a loose piece of movable skin at the end of the penis; it's called the foreskin. Sometimes, parents decide to remove the foreskin, usually a few days after a baby is born. This is called circumcision. If you have your penis circumcised, it still works exactly the same way and is just as clean and healthy as an uncircumcised penis. All penises look different, but it's not anything to worry about."

Years ago, almost all baby boys in North America were circumcised because people thought it would help them to keep penises clean and healthy. These days, we know that soap and water is enough to keep penises clean and healthy, so we no longer circumcise every penis. It really is up to the parents to decide. Sometimes circumcision is done for religious reasons, such as in the Jewish and Muslim faiths. And don't forget that people who don't have a penis need to know this information, too.

Usually, babies assigned male at birth are born with two testicles in the scrotum, or scrotal sac, behind the penis, between their legs (you can be perfectly healthy and fertile with only one testicle). Kids call them "balls" or "nuts" (among other terms) because of their shape. It's fun to point out that most girls have "balls" too. But in girls they're called ovaries, and they are inside the body, on either side of the uterus. The ovaries stay inside the body because the eggs (ova) need to be kept warm. One time in a Grade 3 class, I asked the students, "Why do you think most boys' testicles are outside the body but most girls' ova-

55

TALK
SEX
TODAY

ries are inside the body?" One of the girls suggested, "Because we're prettier?" Testicles and ovaries are also known by another scientific name: gonads.

In most boys, the testicles drop from inside the abdomen into the scrotum at birth, because they have to be kept four to five degrees cooler than body temperature. The scrotum is made of special skin that is stretchable and shrinkable, so that the testicles can be pulled closer to the body to keep them warm, or allowed to move away from the body to keep them cool. That's also why, once toilet training is completed, it's not healthy for children to wear tight underwear to bed every night. As Meg explains, *"You'll make your testicles too hot. That's also why they make pajamas with a deep crotch, so there's room for air conditioning at night. Or you could just sleep in a T-shirt, or nude."* Years ago during a family evening session, we were discussing the importance of keeping the testicles cool and I suggested that if a dad slept nude he would have some of the healthiest testicles in Canada. Right then, one of the kids turned to their dad in the sea of parents and enthusiastically gave him the "thumbs-up" sign.

The testicles make two very important things: sperm for reproduction, and a growth hormone called testosterone. Because the testicles are so important and also so fragile, I stress to kids that it's crucial to keep them safe. Even if someone is just joking around, it's never okay to purposely kick, punch, or hit someone in the testicles. It's also not okay to do "wedgies" (underwear pulled up between the legs).

The testicles are kind of like the brain in that once they're damaged beyond a certain point doctors may not be able to fix them again. The testicular injury to be most concerned about is called a torsion. This is when the blood supply to the testicles (and ovaries, too) gets twisted. In children of all ages, a torsion can be caused by a hit, but it can also happen even when there's no obvious reason. If your child complains of testicular pain or swelling, don't wait around. Go to a doctor right away.

Although twisting of the blood supply to the ovaries is rare, it's important to recognize the possibility. If your child, no matter how young (even a three-year-old), complains of intermittent, intense abdominal pain, nausea, vomiting, fever, or loss of appetite, ask your doctor about an ultrasound.

Sometimes parents feel hesitant to take their child to a hospital or clinic because of testicular pain. Sometimes the child is so shy they'll resist examination. And believe it or not, sometimes *doctors* hesitate because of shyness, or because of lack of experience with torsions. Some doctors might simply give antibiotics, hoping that the pain and fever is caused by an infection. But it never hurts to ask, "Could we rule out an ovarian or testicular torsion?"

Bodies with a penis and testicles usually have two openings between the legs. One opening is the urethra, at the end of the penis, where urine and sperm come out. It's important to explain that everyone's bladder collects urine and is in the same place, just under the skin, above the pubic bone. Most boys have a long urethra so they stand up to urinate. Most girls have a shorter urethra, so they sit down to urinate.

The other opening between the legs is the anus, where stool comes out. I suggest you use stool as the scientific word – among several that could be used – so that if a doctor ever asks for a stool sample your child will know what they're talking about.

It's perfectly appropriate to get a hand mirror and let children have a look between their legs so that they can "be scientists" and know about their bodies. A natural time for this is during their bath, when parents are present to supervise and can make sure that exploration of a sibling's body doesn't occur. Parents should be within earshot at bath time, if not actually present, to protect each child's privacy.

■ BODIES WITH A UTERUS, OVARIES, VAGINA, AND VULVA

I ask young children "If most boys have two openings between their legs, how many do most girls have?" You can imagine the varied responses I get. Somewhere between zero and 17 is the usual range! Many children think that there's only one opening

TALK SEX TODAY

Clitoris
Labia
Urethra
Vagina
Anus

FUN FACT: The vagina is the cleanest opening in the whole body. Seriously! It constantly makes moisture, just like your eyes do. Sometimes the moisture comes out of the vagina during the day and you can see it on the toilet paper; it looks like water during most of the month and like raw egg white when the egg (ovum) is released from the ovary. Sometimes it dries to a yellowish or whitish color on your underwear. That's a good sign that your vagina is clean and healthy. It's kind of like a self-cleaning oven.

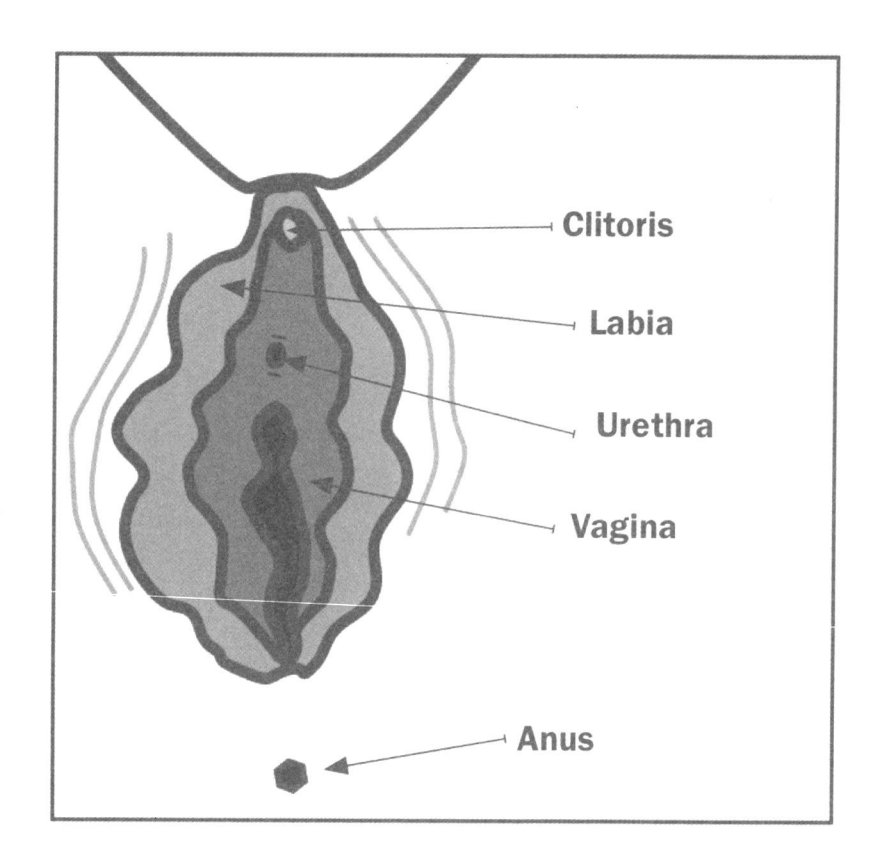

between a female's legs. We, as adults, set them up for this misunderstanding when we tell them that people have either a penis or a vagina. Children then believe that girls have one giant opening between their legs and that everything comes out of it, or they believe that "vagina" is the name for everything between their legs. Indeed, one time during my visit to a Grade 2 class, one of the boys exclaimed, "Did you know that a girl's penis is called a vagina?"

It's much more accurate to say, "Most boys have a penis and most girls have a vulva," referring to the skin between the legs.

The outside skin on a girl's genitals is called the vulva. The vulva is made up of folds of skin called the labia.

Smegma is the name for the white secretions that form between the folds of the vulva and under the foreskin on the penis. Smegma is produced for cleansing and lubrication. It's normal and healthy and nothing to be ashamed about. Children simply need to be taught to wash it away, just like washing behind their ears.

At the front of the vulva, where the folds come together, is a part of the body called the clitoris. The visible part of a clitoris is as big as the end of your baby finger and it can become erect when a person is sexually excited. But the clitoris doesn't "practice" erections like the penis does. The "tickling" feeling that's experienced sometimes is due to extra blood moving into the genital area during sexual arousal. Vaginal moisture may also increase during arousal.

This is a good place to acknowledge that all children are born with the ability to have an orgasm, and genital feelings of sexual arousal may occur in children at a very young age. But kids who aren't educated about these really normal responses can feel shame and guilt. The message we want to give them is that sexual feelings are healthy at every age, but are private. Parents often ask me if what their children are doing (watching TV with their hands down their pants, riding furniture, rubbing a stuffed animal between their legs before bed) is masturbating. The answer is yes, and that's *also* normal and healthy. It's so private, though, that no one can watch you do it, not even a parent. So if a child is masturbating, an appropriate response might be, "**I know that feels good, and I'm glad you are getting to know your body. But you need to do that in private, like in your bedroom or in the bathroom where no one else is around. It's not bad and you're not in trouble; it's just that exploring your body is a private activity.**"

Below the clitoris is the urethra, where urine comes out. Below that is the vagina, where the baby usually comes out. The vagina is about as long as your middle finger and it stretches open by 10 centimetres to let the baby out. The best science for kids to know about the vagina is that, as soon as the baby comes out, it closes again. Whew!

Finally, below the vagina, is the anus where stool comes out.

■ BUT HOW DOES THE SPERM GET TO THE EGG?

When I'm in the classroom, it's not unusual for students as young as kindergarten to ask me, "So if the baby comes out of the vagina, how did it get there in the first place?" Great question! Many children, even at young ages, already understand that in order to make a baby a sperm needs to meet with an egg. There's still a bit of confusion, though, and this information needs to be repeated over and over again. Preschoolers are also very creative in their magical thinking. One time in a kindergarten class I asked, "What do we

> *how does the sperm come out?????*

need from a man's body to make a baby?" One of the students responded enthusiastically, "You need to be romantic!" Another student added, "No, you need a last name!" In another kindergarten class, I was explaining that special cells are needed to make a baby and I asked, "What are these special cells called?" A boy responded, "European cells?"

I could go on for a whole chapter with hilarious examples of children's comments on the topic, but this is how I explain reproduction to young children. First, I say a bit about different ways people become parents and the different kinds of families: **"There are many different ways that people can become parents. For example, some people become parents through adoption. Other people might get the help of a doctor to join the egg and the sperm even outside of the body in the hospital lab. As a result, all of our families are different. Some families have a mom and a dad, some have just a mom or just a dad, some have grandparents raising the kids, some families have two moms or two dads (they're gay families), and some families don't have children at all. Do any of these differences matter? No, a family is a family. In fact, I think these differences are something to celebrate, because they make us all unique."**

I know that's a bit long-winded, but, as a starting place, I think it's important to be inclusive of the different ways families configure themselves.

Which reminds me, one time in a Grade 1 class one of the girls raised her hand and asked, "My mom wrote 'IVF' on my hand this morning. What does that mean?" The teacher told me after that the girl was conceived through in vitro fertilization and her mom wrote that on her hand as a reminder for her to ask me about it.

But back to reproduction. I continue by saying, **"What usually happens when a man and a woman want to make a baby is they put the penis into the vagina to deliver the sperm to the egg. This is called sexual intercourse or 'sex' for short."** I say, **"If this sounds weird or even gross to you, that's totally normal. Mother Nature makes kids feel that way on purpose, because it's only for adults. Not that sex is a bad thing, but it comes with lots of grown-up responsibilities. It's against the law for kids to have sex, and no matter how old people are they never have to have sex if they don't want to."**

As I mentioned earlier, young children are pretty blasé about sex. To them, it's just interesting body science information. And when they *do* have questions about it, they're very mechanical in their thinking, most concerned about the logistics of having sex. For example, a Grade 1 student recently asked me, "Do you have to go to the hospital to have sex, or can you just do it at home?" Another common question for this age group is, "How long does it take to have sex?"

Along with privacy and good manners, teaching about family values and rules when it comes to sex is key. Parents should never be afraid to say, **"In our family, we wait until (we are married…we are a certain age…fill in the blank) to have sex."** Again, children need guidelines and they appreciate reasonable limits.

I always explain to students that the one thing about sex I *can't* tell them is the rules about it. They have to talk to their parents about that, because the rules are different in every family. When time permits, I ask them what they think the rules in their family are. You can imagine the entertaining responses I receive. One kindergarten child suggested that in their family, "You have to use your own bed." A classmate clarified, "But you have to bring them home first and try out a lot of people to make sure they're good." In another class, one of the students reminded me that, "In some families, parents have the kids before marriage so that they can be in the wedding party." Her teacher explained to me at recess that she had just been a flower girl at her parents' wedding.

Speaking of weddings, my younger stepdaughter, Kate, was eight when Chris and I got married. The morning after the wedding, in all of the chaos of an extended family brunch, she pulled me aside and told me that she needed to ask me a question. When I gave her the go-ahead, she asked, "Now that you guys are married, are you going to sex my daddy?" To tell you the truth, I can't remember exactly how I answered, but I'm sure I said something along the lines of, **"Well, yes, having sex is one way that couples show their love and affection for each other."** I asked her if she had any other questions. As I was bracing myself for the next one, she said, "Yah, I'm wondering whether we have to return our dresses or can we keep them?" Whew!

Why was sex invented?

■ TUMMIES ARE FOR BROCCOLI, NOT BABIES

Many young children think that the baby grows in the stomach or tummy, mostly because adults tell them that. Plus, they also notice a pregnant person's belly expanding and assume it's the stomach that is getting bigger with the baby in it. I explain to children that, **"The baby doesn't grow in the stomach or the tummy. If it did, then broccoli and mashed potatoes would come down and bonk it on the head! Instead, it grows in the uterus (womb), a special bag made of strong muscle (so it can stretch)."** It's important to point out that the stomach is an organ about the size of a fist and is located almost under the rib cage. The uterus is a completely separate organ, located below the belly button.

"The uterus stretches bigger and bigger to fit the baby as it grows. It's rude and unfair to call a pregnant person fat. They're not fat; they're just stretched out! After the baby is born, the uterus shrinks back down to original size, just like letting air out of a balloon. The baby is in a water bag (amniotic sac) for protection. So, if the woman falls or is in an accident, hopefully the baby will just bounce around inside and stay safe.

"Because the baby is underwater, it can't breathe or eat through its nose and mouth like we do, so it grows a special cord called the *umbilical cord,* which goes from baby's belly button, which is still wide open, and attaches to the wall of the uterus. The blood vessels in this cord bring oxygen, vitamins, and nutrients from the woman's body to the baby. That's why it's so important to eat mostly healthy things during pregnancy, because food will go straight to the baby through the cord."

As you can imagine, young children have lots of ideas as to what "healthy things" would include. A Grade 1 student suggested, for example, that it wouldn't be a good idea to eat "take-out" during pregnancy. Another warned against hot dogs. And I'll always remember the reaction of an enthusiastic Grade 2 body scientist. He shared that he understood exactly what I meant about the umbilical cord, because his mom told him that being pregnant with him was "torture." When I asked why this was, he explained, "Well, she couldn't have *any* wine!" I then acknowledged that moms make a lot of sacrifices for their babies, to which he responded, "Yah, and you don't know my mom…she *loves* wine." I can usually hold it together when I'm teaching, but the teacher and I had a good laugh about this one.

"When the baby is ready to be born, the strong muscles of the uterus begin to squeeze and relax, squeeze and relax – when this happens, we say the woman is having *contractions*. **Contractions can go on for several hours. To the baby, they feel like giant hugs and actually prepare it to breathe. It's really helpful for the baby to experience this process, which we call labour.**

Eventually, the contractions pop the water bag, making the vagina wet and slippery for the baby to come out. So for most babies, the first waterslide they ever went down was the day they were born. That's pretty fun way to enter the world, right?

Some babies don't come down the waterslide. Instead, they get to come out of the sunroof, which means they are born by a special operation called a Cesarean birth or C-section. In this situation, the

doctor gives the woman some medicine so they can't feel anything, even though they're usually awake. Then the doctor makes a small cut below the belly button to take the baby out of the uterus. Being born through the sunroof is just another really healthy way to be born.

A few minutes after the baby is born and it is breathing properly, someone can take a pair of very clean scissors and cut the umbilical cord near the baby's belly button. Don't worry, it doesn't hurt the baby; it's just like getting a haircut. A few days later, the little piece of cord that's still left on the baby just dries up and falls off (like a scab), creating the baby's very first scar – the belly button. Some people have 'innie' scars and some have 'outie' scars; no one knows exactly why. A few minutes later, when the uterus begins to shrink, the woman pushes out the other end of the umbilical cord (the placenta). And if she has another baby in the future, that baby will grow a whole new cord – we don't recycle those!"

In class, kindergarten and Grade 1 children have lots to share about how they were born, and are fascinated with how the whole process works. Recently, a Grade 1 student couldn't contain his excitement: "I really want to go home now and tell my mom that I went down the waterslide!" he shared enthusiastically.

■ CONDOM AND NEEDLE SAFETY

Kids find condoms all over the place – in parks, at the beach, on the street, and in schoolyards – even in the greatest neighbourhoods. Many parents were raised with negative messages about condoms, but because they see it as a safety issue, they are usually fine with me showing their children examples. Parents sometimes question, though, if it's necessary to teach young children what they're used for. I reply both "yes" and "why not?" You can imagine that if you show a young child something new and tell them not to touch it without explaining what it is, the first thing they'll ask is, "What is that for?" And knowing that children will only absorb what they're ready for at the time, there's no harm in explaining how condoms work at any age. Some kids just won't understand, like one student in a kindergarten class. When I asked at the end of the condom discussion if anyone had any questions, she enthusiastically asked, "Yah, can we see you wear one of those?" And when I ask kids where responsible adults would put their used condom, most often they reply, "In the recycling?"

I like to start my condom talk on a positive note by explaining to children that **"Condoms are clean and healthy when you buy them at the store. They're made of the same rubber (latex) as a doctor's rubber gloves. Of course, men and women sometimes have sex to make a baby. But most of the time, grown-ups have sex not to make a baby but to show their love and affection for one another. And although they want to have sex, they may not want 416 babies.** (There are choruses of agreement and understanding from the kids at this point.) **"So they can wear a condom either over the penis or inside the vagina and, if it works properly, the sperm that comes out of the penis gets caught in the condom instead of going into the body to fertilize an egg. Condoms are also helpful for everyone, because they can stop the spread of germs from person to person."** (Huge sighs of relief emerge from the children and a look of sudden enlightenment appears on their faces).

Now comes the safety: **"When responsible people are finished having sex, they take the condom off and put it in their own private garbage where no one can find it. But sometimes, people are rude and they throw condoms out in parks and at schools and at the beach where children can find them. Condoms don't always look the same. Sometimes they are different colours and sometimes they even have pictures on them. They may look like balloons, but don't pick them up. Instead, report the condom to an adult and they'll remove it in a way that keeps everyone safe. We don't want kids to pick up used condoms because they could get sick from the germs on them. Even if a child has gloves on or is using garbage tongs, it is not their job to pick up condoms and put them in the garbage."**

Although there have been no reported cases of children becoming sick from handling a used condom, we're particularly concerned about the hepatitis viruses, which can survive for a long time in dried human bodily fluid. It doesn't happen as often these days because they have this information, but when I first started teaching several kids reported to me that they had found condoms and tried to blow them up or make water bombs out of them.

Finally, I like to return to the positive message about condoms. **"Condoms are like tissues. They're clean and healthy when you buy them at the store, but have germs on them once they've been used. You wouldn't pick up a used tissue, so don't pick up condoms either."**

For similar reasons, I also show children of all ages examples of syringes and needles. I say, **"Needles are usually clean and healthy, for example, when we get shots from a doctor or a nurse to give us medicine. But if a child finds a needle that wasn't used on them by a doctor or a nurse, would it be a good idea to pick it up and play with it? No.**

TIPS FOR TALKING TO PRESCHOOLERS

Ditch the baby talk: no more pee-pee, wormy, dinky, wieners or boobies. Use scientific names for body parts. Children need to learn appropriate vocabulary for their safety.

Think of teaching your child about sexual health not as "The Talk," but as an ongoing conversation. Have lots of talks, even a two-minute conversation is valuable.

Take advantage of teachable moments. Explain what those monkeys at the zoo are really doing. Tell the truth about relevant family situations (No, Uncle Bryan and Uncle Steve aren't just roommates).

Use books and apps created to help parents just like you. They're lighthearted and fun, they keep children engaged, and they say all the hard stuff for you. A few minutes before bed will allow you to have your preschooler's best attention (they'll do anything to keep you from turning off the light and walking out the door!).

Tell your child a bit more than you think, a bit sooner than you think. Kids are exposed to sex and sexuality at younger ages than we parents like to think, so the key is to stay ahead of the game with accurate information. That way your child will think critically about what they see and hear. Plus, they'll know they can go to you if they have any questions.

Give body science information before they ask. Some kids never ask questions about their bodies, but still need to be educated and protected. And be prepared to repeat yourself 28 times between now and the end of Grade 1.

Instead, report it to an adult and they'll come and remove it in a way that keeps everyone safe." And then the kindergarten students want to share about every immunization they've had and describe exactly what that experience was like for them.

Here's a story that illustrates so well what we hope will happen when children learn condom safety at an early age.

One mom told Meg about waiting at a bus stop with her five-year-old and ten-year-old sons. The younger boy spotted a used condom. The mother said that her heart nearly stopped with panic as she pulled him away, because she didn't know what to say.

Remember that you can't tell a child too much, they only absorb what they need to know at the time. Anything that isn't relevant, interesting or on their radar yet will just go over their head. Trust me.

Don't panic when your child asks a question and you have no clue how to respond. Stay cool, congratulate them for asking such a great question and explain that you need some time to think about a scientific answer. Get back to them after dinner or before bed (or when you get out of the grocery store or when your guests leave…). And if you hate the answer you gave, there's always a chance for a re-do.

No matter how hard or embarrassing your child's questions are, try not to get mad or to act shocked. Start by asking where they heard of what they are asking about so that you know the context, and be proud that they are curious about sexual health. Remember, questions are the most natural opportunity to provide life-saving information. And if your child didn't trust you as a credible source of information, they would ask their friend's older brother. Go you!

You know what they say about practice: Say "penis goes into the vagina to deliver sperm to the egg" over and over again while you empty the dishwasher (in your head, probably). If you can master a few key words or phrases, I promise answering your child's questions on the spot will be way less stressful.

Lighten up. Don't take yourself too seriously and enjoy the funny use of words, mispronounciations and questions. I see many entertaining and invaluable conversations in your future!

Ten-year-old son to the rescue! "Don't touch those, Tyler. People use them to have sex and they can have serious germs on them." The five-year-old said, "Okay. Can I look at your comic now?" The mom, filled with gratitude and admiration, asked her son how he knew that.

"Oh, we learned about that at school in body science," he said, very matter-of-factly.

■ PUBERTY PRIMER

Although I don't typically address puberty with students until the primary years (Grades 2 and 3), I encourage parents to introduce periods and wet dreams to their preschoolers if these topics come up. Often, preschoolers are in the bathroom with a parent when they're menstruating, or they see commercials for pads and tampons on TV. It's not uncommon for them to ask questions, so take advantage of the teachable moments!

■ PRESCHOOL CHECKLIST (K–GRADE 1)

Your preschooler needs to know
- the three private parts of the body: mouth, breasts, and genitals
- that they have ownership of their bodies (basics of consent)
- the scientific words related to anatomy and reproduction (i.e. vulva, penis, testicles, vagina, urethra, anus, uterus)
- that reproduction happens when a sperm joins an egg, usually (but not always) through sexual intercourse.
- that the baby grows in the uterus (not the stomach)
- that the baby is usually born through the vagina
- that families are formed in different ways and are all unique
- not to pick up condoms or needles

Bonus points
- basics about gender stereotypes
- basics about periods and wet dreams

■ RESOURCES

FOR PARENTS

WEBSITES
- www.teachingsexualhealth.ca
- www.seican.org
- www.seicus.org
- www.sexualhealth.com
- www.sexualityandu.ca

Teaching kids sexual consent
- http://goodmenproject.com/families/the-healthy-sex-talk-teaching-kids-consent-ages-1-21/

Understanding children's sexual behaviours
- http://www.tcavjohn.com/products.php

Views of Canadian youth on gender roles
- http://becauseiamagirl.ca/file/2011-BIAAG-Chat-Sheet-on-Canadian-Survey.pdf

FOR PRESCHOOL CHILDREN
(WITH THEIR PARENTS)

APPS
- *Clementine Wants to Know…* www.clementinewantstoknow.com. This app is for preschoolers, primaries, and their parents. Clementine is a precocious six-year-old dynamo with an outsized curiosity about the world around her. When Clementine finds out she is having a baby brother, she embarks on a journey to learn where babies come from and what it's like to be a big sister. Along the way, Clementine explores love and birth. Meg Hickling consulted on this app.
- Birdees (www.birdeesed.com) arms parents with the information and resources to handle tough conversations about sexual education with their child.

BOOKS
- *Boys, Girls & Body Science*, by Meg Hickling.
- *Outside In and See How You Grow*, by Clare Smallman, E. Riddell, and Dr. Patricia Pearse.
- *The Very Touching Book*, by Jan Hindman.
- *What's the Big Secret? Talking about Sex with Girls and Boys*, by Laurie Krasny Brown and Marc Brown.
- *Where Did I Come From?* and *What's Happening To Me?* by Peter Mayle. (Also available on DVD).

Books that break down gender stereotypes
- *10,000 Dresses*, by Marcus Ewert. Bailey dreams about beautiful, magical dresses every night, but during the day no one wants to hear about it. Until a new friend helps Bailey make his dreams of dresses come true.
- *All I Want To Be Is Me*, by Phyllis Rothblatt. A book that reflects the diverse ways that young children express and experience their gender identity.
- *Dogs Don't Do Ballet* by Anna Kemp. Biff is a dog who loves music and moonlight and walking on his tiptoes. Biff also thinks he's a ballerina. But dogs don't do ballet – do they?
- *I Look Like a Girl* by Sheila Hamanaka. Young girls imagine themselves as a dolphin in the sea, a horse on the mesa, a wolf and tiger and "what is wild, in the heart – so I can be me."
- *Interstellar Cinderella*, by Deborah Underwood. A plucky retelling of Cinderella with a fairy godrobot and a princess who dreams of fixing up rocket ships.
- *Jacob's New Dress*, by Sarah and Ian Hoffman. Jacob loves to play dress up, when he can be anything he wants to be. But what Jacob really wants is to wear a dress to school.
- *Little Kunoichi, The Ninja Girl*, by Sanae Ishida. Little Kunoichi is a ninja in training who finds that ninja skills don't come easily. She needs determination, perseverance and hard work to unleash her power.
- *Morris Micklewhite and the Tangerine Dress* by Christine Baldacchino. Morris is a little boy who loves outer space and painting

beautiful pictures and most of all, his classroom's dress-up centre. A story about creativity and the courage it takes to be different.

- *Play Free*, by McNall Mason and Max Suarez. *"Girls can wear pants, boys can wear dresses. None of that should make any messes."* A story of gender expression and acceptance, and a special playhouse where everyone is free to be who they are.
- *Players in Pigtails* by Shana Corey. A fictional account of the All Girls Professional Baseball League formed during WWII, about a girl named Katy who is determined to make it to the big league.
- *Princesses Can Be Pirates Too!* by Christi Zellerhoff. No Girls Allowed? Not only can girls be pirates too, they can do it in a crown and a puffy pink gown.
- *Roland Humphrey Is Wearing a WHAT?* by Eileen Kiernan-Johnson. Roland Humphrey loves wearing pink and sparkles and doesn't understand the "rules" for what boys should like. If girls can like sports and ballet, why can't he?
- *Rosie Revere, Engineer*, by Andrea Beaty. Rosie Revere creates great inventions from odds and ends, and dreams of being an engineer. Afraid of failure, she hides her creations away, until her great great-aunt Rose shows Rosie that the only true failure comes from quitting.
- *Swamp Angel*, by Anne Isaacs. Angelica Longrider, also known as Swamp Angel, can lasso a tornado, drink an entire lake dry, and wrestle a bear in this tall tale set on the American frontier.
- *When the Bees Fly Home*, by Andrea Cheng. Sensitive, artistic Jonathan isn't sturdy enough to help his father with beekeeping, but when a drought hits, the family struggles to make ends meet and Jonathan uses his art skills to save the day.

4. The Bathroom Humour Types

4. The Bathroom Humour Types

■ PRIMARIES (GRADES 2–3)

Meg tells a story that perfectly illustrates the typical reaction of primary-aged children to learning body science. Here it is in her own words.

In a primary family session, I get to the part where I say "and the father puts his penis in the mother's vagina for the sperm to be delivered…" One five-year-old cherub speaks: "Oh my goodness! When I get married I am going to have to tell my wife about this, and she is going to be very surprised!"

"Well maybe she will know this already."

"Oh no she won't, and she's going to be very embarrassed."

"But perhaps she will have had a science lesson like this."

"Oh no, not my wife, I doubt it."

"Well maybe she is here tonight."

Child takes a quick look around and says, "Nah, I wouldn't marry any of these girls."

■ WE LOVE MECHANICAL CURIOSITY

In addition to their very practical approach to body science, a wonderful characteristic that primaries have in abundance is mechanical curiosity. This is the ability to ask without shame or hesitation, "Exactly how does it work?" Meg and I wish that curiosity would last their whole lives! Here's an example: A six-year-old boy was talking to his dad after a body science session and said, "Dad, try to think like a scientist. How did you get your penis off to deliver the sperm to the lady's vagina?"

Here are some most commonly asked questions by primaries that also illustrate mechanical curiosity: "What if you want to do sex but you don't know how?" "Do people lie down to have sex?" "If you want two kids, do you have to have sex twice?" and "What if you have to pee during sex?"

It's so important that we parents welcome these questions and use them as teachable moments. We should treat every question with re-

Does the uteraus have holes so the spirm can enter?

Q. What does the penis do inside the vagina?

spect and grab every opportunity that presents itself to give science and health information. And being lighthearted about it is key with this age group. Enjoy the questions, the misuse of words, the mispronunciations, the misunderstandings – your own as well as your child's.

■ BEWARE BATHROOM HUMOUR

In the primary years, children's jokes tend to centre around underwear and bare bums – a trait that's perhaps not as endearing as mechanical curiosity. Primary kids can make every word in the English language rhyme with pee, poo, and diarrhea. They're fascinated by elimination and their favourite thing to do is to fart. If you think for a moment, you can probably name several friends of yours, even relatives, who are stuck at this level!

We think that children go through this stage of being mesmerized by elimination because they have the digestive system confused with the reproductive system. That gives elimination a huge amount of power. All that giggling, exchanging jokes, rhyming, and constant anal attention is a means of exploring and a reflection of curiosity about sexuality and sexual health.

Sexually immature adults add to the confusion of our children when we tell them that babies grow in stomachs or tummies, and when we say that boys have a penis and girls have a vagina. Some people also say that the woman has eggs and the man has seeds – all related to food and digestion. Naturally, children assume from all of this that a person eats or swallows something to get the baby into the stomach, and many imagine that they'll "poo" the baby out, or vomit or cough the baby up, or the belly button opens.

I'm always amazed by adults who would rather tell children that the doctor cuts a body open to get the baby out than tell them about a vaginal birth. If you had your child by Cesarean, it is perfectly fine to say that, but please don't pretend that that is how *all* babies are born.

Let's be fair to those parents who've done a wonderful job of being open and honest with their preschoolers and primaries, but who still find them rolling on the floor with their friends in response to bathroom humour. Your child is smart; they know what they have to do to be part of a peer group, and this is peer pressure. We also know that kids test words and jokes out on parents to see what kind of reaction they get. Try not to give them one. After hearing the same underwear joke for the 20th time, a parent could simply say, **"I've heard that joke before and I don't find it funny."** Or, **"We're body scientists in our family, so we don't use baby words like that."** Sadly, many adults are stuck at this level and can't talk about any aspect of sexual health without making it into a joke. Slowly but surely we're changing that.

Remember, too, that the stages of sexual development are shrinkable and stretchable. If you have a preschooler and a primary-age child, your seven-year-old has probably dragged your four-year-old into bathroom humour early. Or, if your well-educated four-year-old only hangs out with sexually mature adults, they may skip the primary bath-

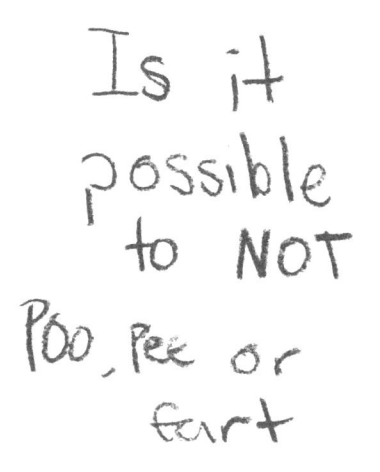

> *Is it possible to NOT poo, pee or fart*

room humour stage altogether.

Now that we have an idea of how primaries approach body science information, the next question is "What do they need to know?" In a perfect world, we would spend time with our primaries reviewing (over and over) everything we've already taught them in their preschool years. But they'll also be ready to learn some new body science, and have lots of great questions too.

■ BE POSITIVE ABOUT PERIODS

Some parents find it shocking that we teach primaries about periods, but we have to remember that some girls start having periods these days as early as age eight or nine. The age of a first period (menarche) in Canada is still closer to 12 or 13, but research tells us it's getting younger by about 6 months every generation. The prevailing theory suggests that this has something to do with hormones and preservatives in our food. Other theories link earlier menarche to a body-weight threshold and childhood obesity. Regardless, it's increasingly important that we talk about periods in an open, positive, healthy way. Whenever the time comes, we don't want a first period to be a scary, traumatic experience like it was for many of us!

Here's how we can explain periods to primary-aged body scientists.

For most girls, at age 12 or 13 (sometimes younger and sometimes older, and that's okay too) the uterus prepares for being grown-up. It does this by making a waterbed inside itself, made of soft skin and a little bit of blood. Each month, when there's no baby in the uterus because an egg hasn't been fertilized, the uterus changes the waterbed and the old one comes dripping out of the vagina. The drips look like blood, but they're mostly water, and it's called "having your period." Scientific words for having a period are "menstruation" or "menses," but all three terms are appropriate to use. We're really glad that most girls get periods because they're a good sign that their bodies are healthy and preparing to reproduce someday, if they want to.

FUN FACT:

Everyone in the world, regardless of gender, experiences the same body changes during puberty except for two: periods and wet dreams. Periods are part of puberty only for people with a uterus, ovaries, and a vagina. So they're experienced mostly by girls. Wet dreams are part of puberty only for people with a penis and testicles. So they're experienced mostly by boys. Every other puberty change happens for all of us!

Most girls get a period once a month and the drips come out for a week or so at a time. It may look like a lot of drips come out every day, but the total is only about the amount of a travel-size bottle of shampoo. During this time *only*, girls need to wear something to catch the period drips. These days, girls and women have lots of options to choose from, including pads, tampons, and special underwear.

Pads are placed in a girls' underwear to catch the drips, and they come in different sizes and thicknesses. They can be disposable (made of soft absorbent paper) or washable (made of cloth). When a disposable pad is full of drips after a few hours or so, a person can just wrap it up in toilet paper and throw it in the garbage can. We don't put pads in the toilet, because they can clog it up. When you change a washable pad, you replace it with a new one and soak the old one in cold water before washing it. That way it won't get stained by the drips. Many washable pads come with a cloth bag that you can use to put the soiled pad in until you can put it in the wash. You can't wear a pad in the swimming pool, because when it soaks up water it'll become really uncomfortable!

As you can imagine, some of the most entertaining comments and questions I hear from primaries come during the discussion of periods and, more specifically, pads. One time as I held up a pad in a Grade 2 class, one of the girls very nonchalantly remarked, "Oh yah, I've seen those. My mom doesn't use them though, she uses coupons."

Tampons work just like pads do, but they're inserted inside the vagina to catch the drips from the inside. Don't worry: the vagina is only as deep as your middle finger so it won't get lost in there. Also, there is a string attached to the tampon that stays partly outside your body, so you can just pull on the string to take it out when it is full of drips. The string can't break off because it's woven through the entire tampon. Tampons are perfectly healthy for people to wear at any age, but it's very important to change it every four to six hours during the day to prevent a bacterial infection. Tampons can be worn for up to eight hours at night when you're sleeping. You can swim with a tampon in, but when you take it out, it's best to wrap it up in toilet paper and put it in the garbage can rather than the toilet. And don't worry; it doesn't hurt at all to put a tampon in. It just takes some practice.

Some companies also make special underwear that you can wear instead of a pad or a tampon; or if you like, you can wear both at the same time.

I was in a Grade 3 class explaining that tampons take getting used

> *How many times does the boys have the sweet dreams in a year?*

to. One of the students agreed: "Yah, just like earrings."

Of course, there are options like menstrual cups and sponges to use during a period, but we'll save discussion of those for the next stage of development.

■ WET DREAMS ARE **HEALTHY TOO**

We don't want people with a penis and testicles to feel left out with all the period talk, so we explain that their bodies practice for reproduction as well.

For most boys, when they're 12 or 13 (sometimes younger and sometimes older, and that's okay too), their testicles start to make sperm for practice. Sometimes some extra sperm come out of the penis when boys are fast asleep at night. Only a spoonful of milky white fluid (semen) comes out and makes a small wet spot on their pajamas or between their legs.

Most boys don't even realize when they've had a wet dream, because it just dries up before they wake up. But we know from research that most people have at least one wet dream in their life, and usually more. We also know that having a wet dream doesn't mean a boy is dreaming about someone cute in his class. It's purely biological and we're glad that most boys' bodies practice for being grown up in this way, because it can help them to reproduce when they're older, if they want to. The super-scientific word for a wet dream is "nocturnal emission." Both terms are appropriate to use.

I respect that everyone has different comfort levels around periods and wet dreams. Trust me, I don't expect a parent to invite their whole family into the bathroom with them while they are changing a pad for fear of missing a teachable moment. But we have to talk openly about these processes as functions that are normal and healthy. They are *private*, of course, but they are not a *secret*. One time, a Grade 4 boy came up to Meg after class and claimed, "My brother is 14 and he's *never* had a wet dream!" She said, "Well, maybe he has, but he didn't feel like telling you; it's private." The boy responded, "Oh, but I'd know, because I sleep on the bottom bunk!" Clearly, he imagined a wet dream as a waterfall coming over the side of the bed.

> *Can girls get wet dreams.*

■ BEYOND PERIODS AND WET DREAMS

It's a good idea to introduce a few basic facts about other puberty changes to primary children. There are two reasons for this. First, they need to know what to expect if they happen to be an "early bloomer," so that they won't be scared or shocked by changes to their body and can share these with you. It's not unusual for kids at this age to start having body odour, pubic hair growth, and breast budding, for example. Of course, some children *do* have what is called precocious puberty and need to be seen by a specialist. If you have concerns that your child's development isn't in the range of normal, talk to your doctor.

Second, there will be early bloomers among their peers and they may be comparing notes. We don't want our kids to feel left out because they don't know what their more informed peers are talking about.

So grab the teachable moments. If an older sibling keeps their deodorant on the bathroom counter, ask your primary child if they know what it's for. It's never too early to teach good personal hygiene habits! Talk about different types of bras while you are shopping for one yourself. And explain that it's normal, healthy, and necessary to gain weight during puberty, if your child voices concerns about their appearance.

What if your boner never leaves.

■ HOT TOPICS: PRACTICE ERECTIONS AND TWINS

Although spontaneous "practice" erections happen long before puberty, primary-aged children start to notice them and often ask, "Why does my penis get hard sometimes?" Good question! Here's how I explain practice erections to primaries.

What's interesting about the penis is that it can only deliver sperm when it's hard. The scientific word for a hard penis is "erection." The reason I'm telling you this is because we know from research that, even before birth, and then several times a day before and during puberty, penises practice erections. That is, at any time – like when a boy is writing a math test, or walking home from school, or even sleeping at night – his penis may get hard for a few moments and then soften again. Practice erections are nothing to worry about or make fun of. They're just a healthy sign that a body is working properly and is practicing for sex and/or reproduction someday.

Primary-aged boys are pretty excited to hear this good news, and often I see them exchanging glances with one another, relieved to hear that they're not alone in their erections!

Primaries also almost always ask me about twins. In fact, they're so fascinated with twins that I could hold their attention for 45 minutes straight discussing the ins and outs of multiples. Common questions about twins include, "Do they come down the waterslide or out of the sunroof?" "How come some twins don't look the same?" "Do twins have their own umbilical cords?" and "Isn't it squishy inside the uterus with more than one baby in there?"

Here's what we can say to primaries about twins: **Fraternal twins (twins that don't necessarily look exactly alike and may even be assigned male and female at birth) happen when two eggs get fertilized by two sperm at the same time, and the babies grow inside the uterus together. Identical twins happen when one egg gets fertilized by one sperm and, soon after the baby starts to develop, the fertilized egg (embryo) splits into two babies. Identical twins look almost exactly alike and are both assigned either male or female at birth. In very rare cases, identical twins don't split all the way and are born joined together at certain parts of their bodies. These are called conjoined twins (we used to call them Siamese twins, but this term is outdated). Depending on where they're joined, parents may ask doctors to separate conjoined twins. But it isn't always possible or safe to do so.**

It's helpful to let kids know that twins each have their own umbilical cord that goes from their belly button to the wall of the uterus – if they didn't, the twins would fight over all the food! How twins come out of the uterus depends on how they're positioned. Sometimes they come out one at a time through the vagina a few minutes apart; sometimes they're born by Cesarean birth; and sometimes one comes out through the vagina and the other comes out by Cesarean birth. Triplets, quadruplets, and other multiples are made in much the same way as twins, either when more than one egg is fertilized by sperm, or when a fertilized egg splits into more than one baby. I also like to remind young children that, although they may have a lot in common, twins have their own unique identities, interests, likes, dislikes, and style.

■ CHILDREN WHO ARE SENSUAL

Some children are born more sensual than others. The sensual ones love being cuddled and want a lot of it. They may show a lot of interest in breasts and genitals – their own and yours! If you aren't a particularly sensual person yourself, this can be challenging. The important thing, though, is to teach appropriate and socially acceptable behaviour. Gently, kindly, remove your child's hands, or pull yours away if your child has placed your hand on their private parts. Explain that this kind of touching isn't appropriate. You could say, **"Those are my private parts and I don't want people to touch me there." Or, "Jacob, it's not appropriate to touch Auntie Susan's breast, because it's a private part. You can sit on her lap as long as that's okay with her, but please keep your hands to yourself." Or, "It's not appropriate for me to touch your penis or kiss your private parts."** You may have to repeat this message firmly, several times.

Just today (no kidding!) I was in a Grade 3 classroom and this issue came up. I had finished the body science lesson and, as I was walking to the door, a boy enthusiastically wrapped his arms around my waist to hug me, and thanked me for coming to their class. The teacher, who was right there, handled the situation beautifully. She gently pulled the boy off me and said kindly to him, "Shane, I know that you love to give hugs to people and you do it because you're friendly and caring. But you just met Saleema. Based on what we've talked about, is it appropriate to hug someone you don't know very well? What would be a more appropriate way you could show Saleema you are grateful for her visit?" Shane thought about it for a minute and, with a huge smile

[handwritten note in margin: Why is the brest a private part?]

on his face, put his hand out to shake mine as he said thank you again. Both the teacher and I congratulated him for his more appropriate sign of affection. It was such a great example of how sensual kids can learn boundaries – with a lot of support and repetition!

Of course, you'll want to stay alert around this issue. Sometimes, a sudden interest in fondling and exploring is an indication that your child has been exploited or abused. Don't panic. Gently repeat the message about privacy and listen for any feedback. If your child responds in a positive way and discloses nothing, you probably don't need to worry.

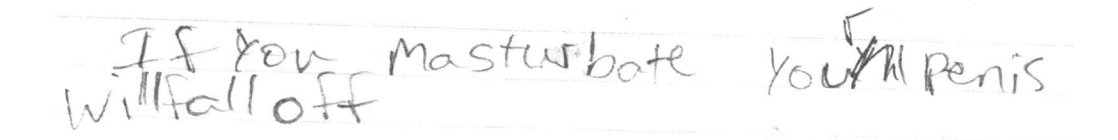

If you masturbate your penis will fall off

■ MASTURBATION DOESN'T STUNT YOUR GROWTH!

Thank goodness there's not one bit of truth to all of those horrible myths we heard growing up about what can happen if you masturbate, or masturbate too much. Not surprisingly, though, these myths are still alive and well today. Many kids, especially sensual ones, enjoy self-stimulating. That's absolutely fine, as long as they also understand about boundaries and privacy. First, some scientific facts. All babies are born with the ability to have an orgasm and babies touch their genitals long before they are born. Most people masturbate (even girls!) because we are *all* born sexual beings. Some children exhibit a great deal of interest in their genitals, others show no interest. It's normal and healthy to masturbate, and it's normal and healthy not to masturbate.

The message needs to be given to children as soon as you can talk and reason with them that touching their body (specifically their genitals) is private. You could say, **"I know rubbing that stuffed animal between your legs feels good, but you need to do that in the bedroom by yourself. You aren't in trouble, it's just a private activity."** We want to give kids positive messages about their bodies and self-stimulation, but we also want to protect them from abuse. Imagine, for example, a scenario with an exploitative babysitter. If you allow your child to masturbate while they're watching TV, or while you're reading them a story, or in public, the babysitter can say, "Hey, that looks interesting. Let me show you how I do it." Just like that, a child can be drawn into an abusive situation.

Thankfully, most parents today no longer punish children for self-stimulating, but saying *nothing* isn't good either. Silence, unfortunately, leaves children open to abuse. So much of what we teach our children about sexual health is about privacy and good manners – touching genitals is healthy, but private.

■ MORE ON PREVENTING SEXUAL ABUSE

Just as some children are more sensual than others, some children seem to be born with very shy personalities. We've all met children who are the life of the party at home with their family, but who are shy at school or in social situations. Other children can be very quiet and seem to be extra sensitive at home, but are active and engaging at school. Parents sometimes suggest that it's because of birth order or gender, but who knows?

I'll be honest; children who are very shy or who are disturbed by learning about sexual health worry me sometimes. And I'm afraid that if the parent gives in to the child's hesitancy to participate and excuses them from body science class, then that child isn't receiving the education that will protect them. What message is the parent sending to their child? And will the child go to them if they have a question? Will the child be able to sort out which stories from the playground are true and which are false? Will they disclose an abusive situation to an adult? Will these children be assertive enough to communicate boundaries as teens? And will they feel comfortable negotiating relationships as adults?

I think parents risk their kids' lives when they shield them from sexual health information. We need to help shy children find their voice, be open, and embrace difficult experiences. We also need to empower them with the skills and confidence they need to keep themselves safe, especially when adults aren't around.

▰ THERE'S ALWAYS A REASON

Shy or not, when children ask questions, there's always a reason. They've either heard something or something has happened – if not, they wouldn't be asking the question. I find a good place to start answering any question is by asking where they heard about the word or activity. Sometimes they're asking the meaning of a slang word, for example, because they heard a friend's older brother use it. As frustrating as it is that your child is learning undesirable slang words and expressions, that's life. Stay calm and explain as scientifically as you can what the word means. If you don't know or if you need some time to think about it, that's okay, too. Just say, **"I'm so glad you about that word. Let me think about how best to explain it to you and we'll talk about it after soccer." Or "That's an interesting word/expression. Even *I* don't know what it means! Let's find out together."**

As difficult as it is to think about, children in the primary years also ask questions because something has happened to them. Meg tells a story that's very sad, but that illustrates the point well:

A mother bravely phoned me in tears one autumn day. She had just discovered that her seven-year-old son had been abused that summer by a 12-year-old boy who lived in their neighbourhood. When she asked her son why he had not told her at the time, he said, 'I tried to tell you, Mom. Remember that day I asked you if guys put their wieners in other guys' bums? You said that only dirty men did that, and I didn't want you to think that I was dirty." This mother discovered the abuse only because her son contracted a serious infection. As parents, we must not let homophobia put our kids in danger.

Of course, the next time your child asks you a concerning question, try not to overreact. Given the story above, it would be totally natural to want to grab your child by the shoulders and demand, "What has happened?" But stay calm, give some basic scientific information, and watch their response. Ask if they have any more questions, and always remind yourself that if they're old enough to ask the question, they're old enough to hear the answer.

If they seem satisfied with your answer (usually they've long moved on to something else!), compliment their curiosity and leave the door open to revisit the topic in the future. You could say, **"If you want to know more about this, be sure to ask me again. I'm really proud of your scientific thinking and I'll always be here to answer your questions."** It's also a good idea to remind your child every now and then that, **"You can always come to me with your questions or share anything that's bothering you. I promise I won't get mad and will do everything I can to make sure you're okay."** We need to make it safe for children to report abuse.

■ BANK ON BEDTIME

With primaries, bedtime is a great time to read a body science book. Let's face it; they'll do anything they can to stop you from turning off the light and walking out the door! This is a good time to hear about worries from school, daycare, or something they saw on a TV. A back rub or foot massage can buy you even more time, as the relaxation almost always provides the safety that's needed to tell deep secrets and hidden fears. It also creates the practice of sharing, which will be especially valuable throughout the teenage years. Trust me on that one!

ALWAYS BE HONEST

As cute and hilarious as our primaries can be when learning body science, The following incident that Meg shares will illustrate this point.

Some parents do not take this stage seriously enough. They do not appreciate that the child is growing up and is no longer a toddler. These parents need to appreciate the mechanical questions, the child's quest for "engineering" information, and the need to grow past the baby talk. Perhaps the following incident that Meg shares will illustrate this point.

In a Grade 3 classroom, when I was talking about the penis delivering the sperm, the children all spoke at once, saying, "Oh, that's having sex," and giggling as usual. One boy, who was also giggling, spoke up and said, "My mom and I have sex all the time." My knees went weak and the teacher's face drained of colour. The boy rushed on to say, "Yeah, we call it sexing when I sit on her lap and kiss her."

The teacher and I were both flooded with relief, and the other students laughed at him, but my point is this: that mother was very, very fortunate. The teacher told me later that the child's statement would have obliged her to call the child protection folks and report the "disclosure," if he had not explained what he meant. It is not the teacher's job to ask for an explanation, or to question the child. After school that day, the teacher telephoned the mother to tell her what had happened. The mother was embarrassed, but explained that she had thought it was "cute" behaviour. She didn't want her boy "to know the facts of life and grow up too fast"! This lad was nine years old and no longer a baby.

I hear shame in that mom's behaviour and great immaturity on

89

TALK
SEX
TODAY

> My Question.
> For the last few years I have had a really big temp. to rub my virgina, I have a really good feeling when I do so, why is this happening?

sex is complicated.

her part. Her behaviour wasn't fair to her son. Not only did she come very close to being the subject of a child abuse investigation, but she left the door open for her son to be teased by the other students, and for stories to go home about her son to the other families. Too many parents assume that because their children are innocent or uninformed, all other children that age are as well. In fact, your child may be the only one who doesn't have good information and a sensible approach in his or her group, from preschool onward.

■ IT'S NEVER TOO LATE!: A FINAL MESSAGE FOR PRIMARIES FROM MEG

If a child's mechanical curiosity is not respected and nurtured, if it is squelched and he is ignored or she is ridiculed, it resurfaces throughout their lives. Sometimes we feel very shy about admitting our curiosity and we repress it, endangering ourselves in the process. Let me tell you about one father who came to his son's Grade 4 class and was quite hostile. He told me he didn't believe sex education should be taught in elementary schools and he told me about some alarming rumours that had been spreading in the community about my presentations. I listened to his tirade, but had no time to reply since the students were waiting.

After the session, the children went for lunch and I asked the father how he felt now. "I never had much more than three years at school," he began, "and if I had heard you when I was nine, my whole #@!!&* life would have been different!" Before I could say a word, he rushed on. "So I've got a couple of questions for you. Why can't we still breathe out of our belly buttons?" Then, in reference to my comments about nocturnal emissions, he asked, "If you never slept, would you fill up with sperm and explode?" Blessings should rain down on this wonderful man forevermore. He asked his questions and he expected me to answer him with all the science that I had. It was one of my proudest moments.

As I tell the children, you never want to run out of questions or stop asking them. And *there is no such thing as a dumb question – not in body science!*

TIPS FOR TALKING TO PRIMARIES

The best way to talk to primaries is the same way you talk to preschoolers. See page 66 for "Tips for Talking to Preschoolers."

■ PRIMARY CHECKLIST (GRADES 2-3)

Your primary child needs to know everything preschoolers need to know, plus
■ the basics about periods and wet dreams as clean and healthy processes

Bonus points
■ more about body changes during puberty

■ RESOURCES

The resources I recommend for preschool children are also appropriate for primary children, so please see the resources list on page 70.

5. The Gross-Me-Outers

5. The Gross-Me-Outers

■ INTERMEDIATES (GRADES 4 AND 5)

Because the intermediate stage of development spans over four years (Grades 4 to 7), I find it helpful to divide these children into two groups: those in Grades 4 and 5, and those in Grades 6 and 7. Although all children in the intermediate stage exhibit similar characteristics in terms of their discomfort and embarrassment talking about sexual health, the nature of what they are exposed to varies, as do their questions as they get older.

There's nothing I teach Grade 6 and 7 students that Grade 4 and 5 students can't hear, and Grade 6 and 7 kids should know everything we teach Grade 4 and 5 kids. But it's helpful to meet each age group's needs more specifically by giving them relevant, age-appropriate sexual health information. For this reason, I'm going to discuss the additional needs of Grade 6 and 7 intermediates separately in the next chapters.

■ GRADES 4 AND 5

I love working with Grade 4 and 5 kids. On one hand, they're beside themselves with discomfort learning about sexuality. They can't believe that I actually teach sex *for a job*, and they write me anonymous notes asking, "Don't you find it gross to talk about sex all day?" or "Do you get paid a lot to do your job?" and "What if I never ever want to have sex? Do I have to?"

On the other hand, they're so glad to see me. They're ready to burst with good questions and are by far the most curious age group when it comes to body science. Luckily, they're very easy to teach once I've gained their trust and we've created a safe environment in which they can learn. That takes about ten minutes.

Of course, in a classroom setting I have a captive audience. But parents find this stage of development challenging because their children just don't want to talk about bodies anymore. They feel frustrated because, despite their efforts to have open conversations with their children growing up and to teach them to be body scientists, their intermediate kids still can't bear to discuss anything to do with bodies, sex, or even puberty with them. Many parents share that they try again and again, but are quickly shut down with comments like, "Yah, Mom, I already know that!" or "I can't believe you're talking about this right now, I'm outta here," or my favourite, "This is *sooo* awkward!" I encourage parents to never give up, because this is such a critical age. Not only is it our last chance to really teach our kids about sexual health and about our values and beliefs that go with that, but they're exposed to so much. They need information to make sense of and think critically about what they see and hear.

Don't worry, at the end of this chapter I'll suggest some ways to keep your intermediate engaged.

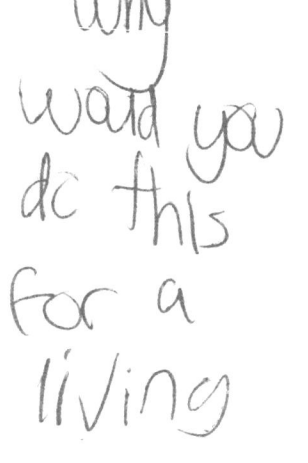

■ HIGH-FIVES FOR **HEALTHY BOUNDARIES**

One of the things that make it difficult to reach out to intermediates about sexual health is their need to develop their own personal boundaries. This can be frustrating, but it's important. It usually manifests as their demand for privacy, first for themselves, then for others. You may have a child who scandalized the neighbourhood with their preschool quest for nudity at all times. Now, overnight, they're not only in the bathroom taking 20 minutes to brush their hair, but the door is locked, dead-bolted, and barricaded. They may feel perfectly comfortable coming in and having a seat while you're on the toilet, but no one's allowed in when they're using the bathroom. Gradually, when intermediates are allowed to develop and maintain their own privacy, they begin to honour other people's need for privacy too. Sexually mature people know their own boundaries and also respect the boundaries of others.

Sadly, this is also the age group that is most often sexually abused – with profound consequences. If children aren't effectively supported after abuse, they tend to go in one of two directions. The first is to build so many personal boundaries around themselves that they never have healthy, joyful, fully satisfying adult relationships; the second is to develop no boundaries at all, either for themselves or anyone else. For example, one time a child told me that they couldn't bring friends home after school, "because my dad sits on the couch watching TV in his underwear." When the child complained, her dad replied, "It's my couch, my house, my television, and my privilege to wear whatever I like." This is an adult who is immature. A mature adult would put the child's needs first and honour the child's quest for privacy. It's the child's home, too, and they need to experience respect for themselves at home before they can learn to respect the privacy of others.

Here's another example of poor boundaries. A Grade 4 child shows up at school wearing a T-shirt that says, "Wine me, dine me, 69 me." Whoever bought the shirt and allowed them to wear it has poor boundaries, to say the least. Not only is that adult disrespecting society's boundaries, but they're violating the child's right to be safe. That child is being set up for judgment, and for some hurtful questions and possible teasing at school. They're also vulnerable to abuse or exploitation. Thankfully, I've only come across that kind of extreme inappropriateness one time in almost 20 years of teaching. More commonly, I see children in Grades 6 and 7 wearing shirts advertising alcohol. In fact, it's become trendy for girls to wear shirts with the Jack Daniels or Budweiser logo on them. Some parents are too busy to notice what their children are wearing to school, some older children change once they get to school so their parents don't see their clothes, and some parents are just clueless.

This makes me both angry and sad. Part of me wants to confront and challenge them. But many of these adults haven't had an opportunity to develop appropriate modesty and boundaries. Sadly, when they were younger, their parents were probably immature too. It all becomes an unhealthy cycle. Children *need* parents and siblings who respect boundaries.

As parents, we need to be clued in to our kids' boundaries, even if they don't express these directly. If a child or teen walks by a parents' room as they're changing and closes the door as they pass, that's a message that they no longer wish to see them nude. We know that sleeping nude is healthy, but covering up in "public" areas of the house is probably a good idea. Remember, whoever says "no" rules. If one person in the family (parent or child) is uncomfortable, we need to respect their need for boundaries and privacy. If no one respects privacy at home, then children don't expect it outside their homes.

Unfortunately, as I've noted, many adults are stuck at this intermediate stage of development because of abuse and lack of respect they suffered when they were young. Others may be stuck in the shy, embarrassed stage because they grew up in homes that may have been physically nurturing, but totally repressed around sexual health. It is really hard to grow beyond the maturity level of your parents, your school, and/or your society.

▌ BEYOND S-E-X

When we teach young children about reproduction, it's important they understand that sexual intercourse is the most *common* way that a man and a woman get a baby, but it's not the only way. Many people become parents through adoption or with the help of a doctor. As a result, all families are unique.

Preschoolers and primaries understand and celebrate these differences without having too many questions about reproductive technologies. Intermediates, on the other hand, have lots of questions and need some additional information about how technologies like intrauterine insemination (IUI), in vitro fertilization (IVF), and surrogacy work. I find that giving examples of how and why these procedures may be used is the most interesting way of explaining them. Here's what I might say:

"**If a single woman wants to become a parent, she may decide to adopt a baby. Or, she can ask a special doctor to put sperm from a sperm donor inside her uterus, in the hope that an egg cell gets fertilized. This procedure is called 'intrauterine insemination,' or IUI.**"

Here's another example that teaches not only about IVF, but also about gay relationships and surrogacy. (I'm careful to stress that it is not just gay people who use these technologies; anyone can.)

> *Could people have babies without any sex?*

> *Do you get paid for donating sperm*

"**If two men in a (gay) relationship want to become parents, they may do that through adoption. Or, they can ask a special doctor to take sperm cells from one of the dads and egg cells from an egg donor, and mix them in a petri dish in a hospital lab. After a few days, when the eggs have hopefully been fertilized by sperm, several of those eggs will be placed in a woman's uterus in the hope that a baby (or babies) will grow. This procedure is called 'in vitro fertilization,' or IVF. The woman who carries the baby for the dads is known as a surrogate, or gestational carrier.**"

Explaining these different ways that people can become parents is important not only to answer questions intermediates have about reproduction. It's equally if not *more* important that we *normalize* the different ways people can become parents. In doing so, we celebrate that all families are unique – some families have a mom and a dad, some families have just a mom or just a dad, some families have grandparents raising the children, and other families have two moms or two dads (gay families). Every family and every relationship deserves respect.

Parents can use this discussion as an opportunity to remind their intermediates about the importance of always talking and acting in a way that reflects this. I say "remind" because my hope is that parents have taught their kids from day one that differences – including sexual expression, gender identity, and sexual attraction – are to be celebrated.

■ CREATING A CULTURE OF INCLUSION

I remember being in a Grade 7 classroom about 15 years ago talking about the importance of showing respect for all relationships. Specifically, we were having a discussion about the importance of not using homophobic words or expressions like, "That's so gay!" with the word "gay" being used to mean "stupid, dumb, weird, or lame." One of the boys asked, "But what if there are no gay people in the room. Then can I say it?" I explained that homophobic language is not just offensive and hurtful to gay people, *anyone* can be affected in a negative way. Plus, you can't tell by looking at someone if they are gay, so it would be impossible to know if there were gay people in the room. He countered by saying, "Oh I can tell." I replied, "Really? How?" To which he responded, "Come on, Saleema. You know all those guys who wear Lululemon."

I'm happy to report we've come a long way since then in terms of challenging stereotypes of gay people, and helping people (of all ages) to understand that homophobia (and transphobia, racism, sexism, and ageism, for that matter) is not okay. Preschoolers and primaries have no problem with this. Intermediates, teens, and even some adults also agree for the most part, but sometimes use homophobic language without even realizing it. The phrase "That's so gay!" and variations of it are still part of kids' everyday language to some extent and, unfortunately, the media reinforces the normalcy of (or increases their desensitization to) this language. Some kids say to me, "Oh, Saleema, relax!

We don't mean anything bad by it; that's just how we talk! My uncle's gay; I love gay people!" My response is simple. Regardless of our intention or our beliefs about homosexuality, homophobic language is never okay. Period.

Even more disturbing is when boys call each other "gay" or "fag" as an insult, with "gay" meaning "weak," "girlie," and "wussy." In fact, this is the worst insult you can give a guy, a perfect example of how gender stereotypes in our society shape what's acceptable (and what's not) depending on whether you are a boy or a girl. From the day they are born, gender stereotypes teach boys that they should be tough, strong, manly, and into girls in order to be a "real guy." Any variation from this unrealistic expectation is interpreted as weakness. This is incredibly unhealthy for our boys, and damaging to their relationships and to our society in general.

Also unacceptable is slang language that's offensive and disrespectful to intersex and transgender people. The most common example used by young people is the term "he/she." We need to help children and teens understand the impact that this cruel language can have on others, especially the marginalized.

[handwritten: I think that it is OK to be homosexual]

Because most kids get this, I encourage them to always call a person out on their use of disrespectful language, comments, or jokes. I suggest that they use a very strong, assertive voice to make simple "I" statements, such as, **"I don't like it when you talk like that," or "I find your language offensive," or "I don't think that joke is funny."** "I" statements work well because no one can argue with our feelings. We have a responsibility to respond in some way, though, because not responding sends a message that we don't care, or that we think how they are acting or talking is okay.

Teaching kids basic assertiveness skills in the intermediate years is an extremely valuable way to help them deal with a range of tough situations beyond homophobia, such as bullying, friendship chal-

■ MORE ABOUT SEX? THERE'S MORE?!

Intermediate children hear so much about sex, mostly in the media and on the Internet. They don't have the knowledge or experience, though, to make sense of what they see and hear, and often make inaccurate conclusions about what sex is really like. They try

> *[handwritten note: why do people even want to have sex]*

so hard to put things together for themselves, and while their attempts are admirable, without factual information they can be dangerous. For example, an intermediate child may hear of adults "sleeping together" as a way to get pregnant. They also have lots of good questions about the mechanics of sex. "Do people have to take their clothes off to have sex?" "Where do people do it?" "How long does it take?" All of these questions deserve scientific answers.

When we teach children about the mechanics of sexual intercourse, we also have to teach healthy boundaries. Intermediates students are relieved when I tell them that it's against the law for kids to have sex, so it's nothing they have to worry about anytime soon. In fact, no matter how old they are, they never have to have sex if they don't want to. You should see the look of relief on their faces! Of course, we don't want kids at any age to think that sex is bad or scary. We've known for years from research that fear-based, problem-focused sex education simply doesn't work.

For this reason, I always follow up by saying something like this:

"Just because it's against the law for kids, we don't want you to think that sex is a bad thing. In fact, in most circumstances, like between two adults in a healthy, consenting relationship, sex is great. It's not only a way that reproduction can happen, but even more often it's a way for people to show love and affection toward each other. Sex also *feels* good. Mother Nature makes it pleasurable, otherwise no one would want to have it and most of us wouldn't be here! Sex will probably be a great part of your life someday, but it comes with lots of responsibilities, so it's a better idea to wait until you're at a time in your life when you can handle them."

When I ask intermediates what these responsibilities are – by the way, I am careful to not use the word "consequences" as it has a negative connotation – they tell me, "Well, you could get a baby and you could get a disease." We talk about how an unplanned pregnancy would impact a person's life at any age, and what it would mean for their future. As parents, it's also important to discuss the emotional aspects of a sexual relationship with our intermediates. And we need to give some basic information about Sexually Transmitted Infections (STIs).

■ STIs DON'T NEED TO BE SCARY

Although we have gone back and forth in the past, the terms STI (sexually transmitted infection) and STD (sexually transmitted disease) are interchangeable. I prefer to use the term STI because "infection" sounds less intimidating than "disease." It also allows a discussion of bacterial infections that can be cured versus some diseases that cannot.

When discussing STIs, parents of intermediates don't need to go into intricate detail about the 50-plus we know about, or into the related signs and symptoms, unless our kids have specific questions. It's more helpful to start by stressing that children don't need to worry about these infections because kids aren't doing anything that could put them at risk. That is, these infections aren't passed or transmitted by hugging, holding hands, sharing food and drinks, or even kissing. Again, we need to be careful to put things into perspective for our intermediates so that we don't scare them unnecessarily. We also have to explain that STIs can affect anyone, regardless of age, gender, sexual attraction, or economic background.

Some babies are born with an STI, and some people contract an STI in ways that have nothing to do with sex (for example, from sharing needles during drug use). Most commonly, though, STIs are passed through sexual activity in one of two ways. Some are passed through the exchange of bodily fluids such as blood, vaginal fluid, and semen (the fluid that carries sperm). Other STIs are passed by skin-to-skin genital contact. Again, that doesn't include holding hands, hugging, or kissing; we're referring to *genital* contact between people. I find it helpful to give intermediates examples of these two kinds of transmission:

"Let's say that a man and woman are having sex, and the man has an STI (although women can have them and pass them on, too) that's passed through bodily fluids. That means the fluid from his penis (semen) is infected as well. If infected semen gets inside a woman's vagina and she has a cut or tear in the vaginal tissue (which can often happen), that's an entrance point for an STI to get into her body."

Or **"If two people are lying naked together with genitals touching and one of them has an STI that can be passed that way, the infection can be transmitted."**

The next question we need to ask our intermediates is, **"So how would a person know if their partner has an STI? Can you tell by looking at them?"** I'm always impressed when students know that the answer is "no" and suggest that partners would have to have an honest, open conversation about their sexual health history. But we can't guarantee our partner is telling the truth, because there's still a lot of shame and stigma about STIs in our society. Also, many STIs are asymptomatic, meaning that they don't have symptoms. Someone could look totally healthy and feel totally healthy, but not know that they have an STI. Knowing this, responsible adults would have the conversation and then both go to a doctor to get tested for a range of STIs, *before* they enter a sexual relationship. It's also worth mentioning that if someone doesn't feel comfortable or is too embarrassed to get STI testing, maybe they aren't ready for sex. I'll say more about being ready for sex in the chapters about Grade 6 and 7 students.

The good news is that other than keeping our genitals to ourselves, we can prevent the spread of at least some infections through the use of condoms. If you haven't already, I recommend showing your intermediate children samples of both an external (male) and an internal (female) condom, not only so they can recognize them on the ground, but also to enhance their understanding of how condoms work. Review how they prevent pregnancy. But also explain that if condoms work (which they usually do if they're used properly) they can prevent the spread of STIs that are passed through the exchange of bodily flu-

> *How many infections are there?*

ids. However, because condoms don't cover the entire genital area, they can't prevent the spread of STIs passed through skin-to-skin genital contact.

More good news is that STIs that are bacterial infections (such as gonorrhea, chlamydia, and syphilis) can be cured with antibiotics. Viral infections *can't* be cured, but doctors have medications they can give to patients to manage the symptoms of some viral STIs. We also have vaccines that can protect people from some STIs, such as human papilloma virus (HPV) and hepatitis B. The body can also cure some viral infections on its own.

Again, we want to achieve a balance with intermediates. We need to help them understand the very real and sometimes serious outcomes of a sexual relationship, but STIs *aren't* a death sentence. We shouldn't and don't need to focus too much on these responsibilities with intermediates; the vast majority of them would be willing to sign a written contract saying they are never having sex! We merely need to reassure them that it's totally their choice whether or not they ever have a sexual relationship, although they may change their mind when they get older.

That reminds me of one mother who told me about her nine-year-old's very typical reaction to body science class. When the mom asked her son, "What did you learn?" he replied, "Mom, the grossest thing, you know how the man puts his penis in the woman's vagina?"

"Yes, but it's really not gross," replied the mom.

"No, Mom, the grossest thing is…some guys like it!"

ADDING TO UNDERSTANDING ABOUT PREGNANCY

Much like primaries, intermediates are fascinated by pregnancy and childbirth and have lots of great scientific questions as they try to make sense of everything. When learning about the baby growing in the uterus, a common question is, "But can a boy have a baby?" Ten years ago, I would have said, "No, because boys don't have a uterus. They have nowhere to grow the baby." Now, I use this question as an opportunity to distinguish between sex assigned at birth and gender identity. We know that at least one man has had two babies. This was possible because he is transgender. He was assigned female at birth, but transitioned to male as an adult. Although he asked doctors to alter the outside of his body physically during this process, they didn't remove his uterus. So he still has a place to grow a baby.

The popular term "lost a baby" is another confusing expression for intermediates on several levels. One girl asked her mother, after hearing family gossip, where Mrs. Jones had *lost* her baby. Her mom replied that Mrs. Jones had lost it at the hospital. Later, in tears, the girl asked why Mrs. Jones hadn't gone back to find her baby, and begged her mom to "never stop looking for me if I get lost."

Many children hear about miscarriages through family gossip or everyday conversations among families and neighbours. Emergency-type hospital TV shows are also incredibly graphic, but not always medically accurate.

First, I like to suggest to kids that they may not have received good information. Then I'm honest with them. Sometimes we know why a woman miscarries. For example, we know that substance abuse and smoking increase chances of miscarriage. Kids also bring up poor nutrition, violence, accidents, and a woman being sick herself. I stress how important it is for a pregnant woman to make sure her body is as healthy as possible, so that hopefully her baby can be healthy as well.

It's important not to let children leave the discussion, though, thinking that all pregnancy tragedies result from carelessness. Doctors and scientists don't always know why some anomalies occur, and there are still many mysteries to be solved when it comes to conception, pregnancy, and birth. For whatever reason, Mother Nature (or whoever you identify with in your family) knows the baby (or embryo) wouldn't survive outside the uterus and ends the pregnancy. Luckily, most women who have miscarried are able to have a baby in the future.

> *How long are you pregnent for?*

I find that intermediates often confuse the concept of a miscarriage with abortion. Many of them have heard of abortion. In fact, a Grade 4 boy asked me just the other day, "Isn't there a way people can cancel the baby if they're not ready for it?" I simply respond that the fertilized egg can be surgically or medically removed from the uterus to end the pregnancy.

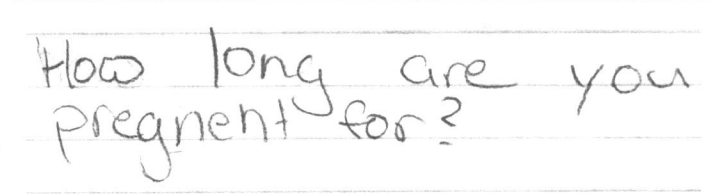

■ EVERYTHING THEY DON'T WANT TO KNOW ABOUT PUBERTY (BUT STILL NEED TO KNOW)

I define puberty as a time in a person's life between the ages of eight or nine, and 17 or 18, when their body changes from being a child to an adult. Lots of different changes, both physical and emotional, happen to a person during puberty. It's important to emphasize to intermediates that, although every person in the world experiences mostly the same body changes, those changes happen at different times for different people. This is a good thing, because it means that an individual's body develops at exactly the right rate for them. These differences also make us unique!

Intermediates are in the thick of puberty and have a huge need for information about their changing bodies and emotions beyond the obvious observation that they are turning into larger humans. But rather than wait for children to start puberty, parents would ideally talk about these changes long before they happen. Even preschoolers ask, "Will I have bigger boobies when I grow up?" or "Will I have hair down there?" or "Will I need a tampon when I'm bigger?" A simple "yes" is a great answer, and is usually enough for young children. But the easiest way to start these conversations is when questions come up. Puberty can be a time of incredible angst for preteens. Indeed, just the other day I asked a Grade 5 class, "What happens during puberty?" and one of the students replied, "Everything falls apart?" Recently, a Grade 6 student asked me, "When does puberty strike?" It's great to be able to offer intermediates some comfort about their growing bodies, and to normalize these changes when they feel no one else understands. Here are some important puberty changes we should discuss with intermediates:

■ BOYS HAVE BREASTS TOO

Not surprisingly, many of the questions that intermediates ask centre around breasts: "When should they start growing?" "When should I start wearing a bra?" "Do I have to wear a bra?" "Is it normal for my boobs to hurt sometimes?" "Why do guys love them?"

I like to let students know right off the bat that every breast is unique, even on the same body. One breast will start growing before the other, one will grow faster than the other, one will be a different size and shape than the other, and one will point in a different direction than the other. It's also helpful to point out that size doesn't matter. Adult women have breasts to feed babies, if they choose, and smaller breasts make just as much milk as larger ones. I also like to point out that real adult breasts are not perfectly symmetrical, perky watermelons on a person's chest like we see on TV, and in movies and magazines.

In terms of when to start wearing a bra, it's different for everyone. Some girls start wearing bras in elementary school, others not until high school. Some girls choose never to wear a bra, and that's okay too. It really depends on what's comfortable for them. I think it's worth pointing out to boys that the decision to wear a bra or not wear a bra can be very difficult for girls, so it's never okay to make fun of someone because they are or aren't wearing one.

Boys develop breasts too during puberty. They need to know that this is normal and that when their rib cage grows to adult size, they'll spread out and not be so noticeable. It's important for all intermediates to know that they may feel little bumps underneath the skin in the breast area, and they're nothing to worry about. They're growing bumps, "nodes" we call them, and they'll come and go from time to time due to hormone changes in the body during puberty. Of course, we don't want a puberty-aged child to feel these healthy bumps and worry that they have breast cancer. Breast tenderness is also related to hormonal changes during puberty and is totally normal.

For the record, let your intermediate know that not "all" boys are obsessed with big breasts. What people find sexually attractive varies greatly, and it's inaccurate to assume all men are into them – just like it's inaccurate to assume that *all* women are into facial hair, right?!

▰ VOICE CHANGES

Voices change during puberty – girls' voices too. Sometimes it happens slowly over several months, and sometimes it seems to happen overnight. Much like breast growth can make girls feel self-conscious, boys can feel uncomfortable that their voice sometimes goes higher before it goes lower. This can result in a boy sounding like an out of tune clarinet for a few months. I stress that it's not cool for girls to make fun of their brothers during this time, and that it's important to respect how difficult this can be. That's another good reason why I always teach boys and girls together – so that they understand and respect each other's experience of puberty.

■ THE HAIR "DOWN THERE"

It's no shocker that body hair grows in during puberty. In fact, some children begin growing underarm hair and pubic hair as young as Grade 2, others not until high school. It doesn't take children long to notice that women (and men as well) often remove their body hair. Point out that this is a personal choice; there's no health reason for it. In North American culture, the majority of people remove body hair, while in many others people don't see the need.

That being said, if your child shares that they'd like to start to shave or wax, don't let it become a power struggle. In our increasingly hairless society, many girls at this age feel really self-conscious about hair under their arms, on their legs, and even on their face and forearms. If this is the case for your daughter, talk to her about hair removal options. And then help her with whatever the two of you choose is the best option for her. For example, buy her a good razor and teach her how to shave properly. This can be difficult for parents to get their heads around, but seriously, don't sweat the small stuff. There will be far more important struggles to come, and besides, girls already have enough chipping away at their self-esteem, body hair doesn't need to be one of those things!

Intermediate children have both a fascination and anxiety around pubic hair. They ask me questions like, "Why does hair grow between the legs?" "If you dye your hair green, will your pubic hair turn green too?" "How come pubic hair never gets too long?" and "Do you lose your pubic hair when you get old?" Scientifically, kids need to know that pubic hair is not just for decoration. Its purpose is to protect the genitals, much like we have eyelashes to keep germs out of our eyes, and we have hair in our nostrils to keep germs out of our nose.

But I think the fascination about pubic hair comes from children at a young age learning that many people have their pubic hair removed or shaped. They see photos in magazines, and sandwich boards outside of stores advertising deals on "Brazilians" and "manscaping." They also see women in real life at the beach, and it's not difficult to notice that there's no hair sticking out of their bikini bottoms. Some kids are exposed at this age to pornography online and see pretty clearly that neither the women nor the men have pubic hair (or any other body hair for that matter).

I stress to intermediates that pubic hair is important, but people can choose whether they want to remove or shape it. With teenagers, again it's a matter of not sweating the small stuff. If your teenage daughter is self-conscious about her pubic hair protruding from her swimsuit, talk to her about removal options such as waxing or laser. Shaving pubic hair isn't a good idea as the skin is very sensitive in the bikini area and can easily develop an itchy and painful rash. There's a difference, though, between waxing the bikini line and a Brazilian, which removes all pubic hair. I'd say Brazilians are a no-go for preteens and teens.

▪ THE SCIENCE OF SWEAT

When people get hair on their body, they naturally start to sweat more. This is a good thing, because sweating helps keep our bodies cool. But we need to explain to puberty-aged children the "science of sweat." Here's how I do it.

"When sweat comes out of your body it's clean and odourless. But within seconds after you start sweating, bacteria from all over (insert your neighbourhood), and even some from (insert your neighbouring neighbourhood), come and live in your sweat. Bacteria stink, so you have to wash them off your body every single day, especially in the genital area, even if you don't feel sweaty, even if you don't have gym class, and even if it's cold out."

Without fail, immediately after I say this, a Grade 5 boy will stick his head in his shirt and say, "What are you talking about, Saleema? I haven't showered in a few days and I smell fantastic!" I then have to break the news to them that they're immune to their own stink. They're so used to it, so they can't smell themselves anymore, but they need to trust me, they don't smell very good!

Intermediates have lots of questions about deodorant. I suggest they talk to their parents about a natural kind to buy, if they feel they

FUN FACT:
It takes three years after the onset of puberty for testicles to grow to adult size. But the crucial science that boys are often missing is that it takes *eight to ten years* after the onset of puberty to grow their penises to adult size.

need it. There are lots of good ones on the market now that are a better option than antiperspirants with potentially harmful chemicals in them. (The jury is still out on this, but why take the risk?) We also need to remind our children that deodorant should be put on right after a bath or a shower before the bacteria get to us. I always giggle to myself when I see a group of Grade 7 boys coming out of the gym changing room in a cloud of Axe or Tag spray antiperspirant. They may as well just take their glue stick from their desk and glue the bacteria to themselves, because they're going to smell just as bad by the end of the day!

It's also crucial for intermediates to understand the importance of washing their clothes on a regular basis. Not that I would ever want to create extra laundry for a household, but underwear and socks need to go in the wash every day. The smell test is also important for shirts that touch the underarms directly, and gym strip should be taken home from school to be washed at least once a week. These good personal hygiene habits are important not only so that we smell good, but also so that our bodies aren't at risk of infections and rashes as a result of uncleanliness.

> *why dose mom say i smell bad when i Don't smell it?*

■ THE INCREDIBLE SHRINKING PENIS

I get tons of anonymous questions from intermediate boys asking, "Is it possible for your penis to shrink during puberty?" and "What's the world's longest penis?" What they're *really* asking is, "What's the world's *smallest* penis, because I think I've got it." You probably didn't have to buy this book to learn what I'm going to say next, but I'll say it anyway. Preoccupation with penis size lasts a lifetime!

Because kids are often exposed to pornography and therefore see the "stars" with giant penises, it's a good idea to explain to them that no one has a giant penis in real life. In fact, when penises get erect, they're all about the same size (between five and seven inches long, but sometimes smaller and sometimes bigger, and that's just fine too). The truth is, the penis fills up with blood to get erect. If you had a humungous penis and it filled up with blood, you'd faint and it wouldn't do you any good. The porn industry uses a variety of methods to make penises look "larger than life", including drugs injected directly into the penis, penis "add-ons" or extensions, pairing a petite female actor with a large male actor, manipulating camera angles and lighting, and so on. In other words, the super-sized penises in pornography aren't always "real."

Just to add to everyone's scientific knowledge here, flaccid or soft penises can be all different sizes – long, short, fat, thin, even curved. As long as they work without any discomfort, they're fine. And remember that the penis is designed to deliver sperm and that you only need about two inches to do that. Anything you get after that is a bonus.

> *If you have a small penis will that effect your relationship.*

This is a perfect time to talk with your child about the hugely distorted and exaggerated images of the human body in media, and about how the media manipulates and shapes our perceptions of what is beautiful, handsome, and attractive. Grab this teachable moment with gusto, respect your child's ideas and, most importantly, maintain a sense of humour.

■ PARTY ON WITH YOUR PERIOD

I don't think there is much need to belabour the intricacies of having periods with young people. Instead, I concentrate on the health of the process. The lining or endometrium of the uterus is shed each month; I don't use phrases such as "the uterus cleans itself" because I think such phrases suggest that it's dirty. As long as there is no infection, menstrual flow is clean. Of course, we have to wash our vulva daily, or bacteria can cause the flow on the outside to have an odour.

Another misconception about periods is that the unfertilized egg comes out with menstrual flow. In reality, it begins to dissolve 12 hours after it comes out of the ovary. It's pure protein and the body simply reabsorbs it, usually from the abdominal cavity. The egg may never enter the fallopian tubes. Another common misunderstanding, usually from the ridiculous and outdated filmstrips we saw when we were at school, is that menstruation is connected to ovulation, and vice versa. The truth is that most people with a uterus miss ovulating two or more months a year. They still have their periods, but that's not proof that they've ovulated. And sometimes a person is ovulating, but not menstruating. When a person begins to menstruate, they can be very irregular. It usually takes two to four years to become regular and some people never become regular. For the most part, whatever your body does is healthy for you.

Cramps and painful periods can be annoying and even debilitating for some (but not all) at this age. I suggest that a heating pad on the lower abdomen may ease the discomfort. I also recommend that people keep their bodies moving if they have cramps, because this increases blood flow to the uterine muscles and helps them to relax. So when students ask if they can be excused from gym class because of period cramps, the answer is "Nope!" Of course, severe cramps may be helped with medications like ibuprofen or prescription medication.

Once girls start getting used to having a period, parents can also introduce different methods (beyond pads and tampons) of catching the menstrual flow, such as menstrual cups and sponges.

A menstrual cup is a small plastic cup-shaped container that's placed inside the vagina to catch period drips. Every few hours, a girl can empty it into the toilet, rinse it with warm water, and place it back in the vagina. A cup can be worn for up to 12 hours at a time, it can be sterilized between periods, and it can be reused for years (which means it's not only economical, but great for our planet too!). Some are made of latex, and the DivaCup is made of silicone, which means it can be used by women who are allergic to latex. Although not super popular among young girls, a natural sea sponge can also be placed in the vagina to catch period drips. It can be rinsed and placed back in the vagina every few hours, and it can be reused for years, as long as it's sterilized properly between periods to prevent a bacterial infection. Some companies, such as Lunapads, also make special underwear that you can wear to catch period drips.

Let your daughter know that people often use a combination of pads and tampons or cups, depending on how heavy their menstrual flow is, and whether it's day or night, and what is most convenient at the time. At the end of the day, which method to use is a personal choice and all the methods are painless and safe to use at any age.

It's too bad that, even today, attitudes about periods are so negative. People still refer to having a period as "the curse" or "being on the

> *Why is being flat chested bad or not sexy?*

rag." No wonder girls dread getting it! Students think I'm joking when I tell them that in many cultures a first period is cause for a big celebration. For our North American kids, a "First Period Party" may sound like a totally weird idea, but it's a beautiful rite of passage that's been recognized throughout history all around the world. I challenge you to suggest a First Period Party to your newly menstruating child. Or at least brainstorm other ways to celebrate this huge milestone in their life.

■ EMOTIONS: THE SADS, MADS, AND GLADS

Children can learn how to manage their emotions during puberty, but they need our support. We can to normalize this time of emotional intensity and help them develop coping skills. I tell kids, **"It's normal to have hormone attacks and to feel as if you're out of control, but it's *not* okay to punch holes in walls or to try to murder your little sister at dinner with your fork. It's not her fault that you're in puberty and she deserves to live a full life!"**

We call these normal, healthy mood swings the "sads, mads, and glads." The sads are when you become hypersensitive; every little thing bothers or worries you, and you cry but don't know why. You feel alone and that no one likes you, that you're ugly, and you hate your parents. I always try to give parents a heads up about this last aspect of the sads. Don't take it personally, and despite what your child may say, this dislike has nothing to do with your job, your interests, your looks, or just being uncool. *All* parents face intense dislike from their children at one point or another: if we didn't, we wouldn't be doing our job! It's the hormones talking, and if we're being honest, there are times when we parents don't like our kids much either. Stay calm, rise above it, and take a moment to remember your own rebellious thoughts at that age.

Of course, there's a fine line between what might be considered normal hormonally-induced puberty blues and clinical depression that needs serious attention. Don't leave your child for weeks to figure it out on their own. Trust your gut. If they don't seem to snap out of the sads after a few days, step in and offer support. And don't hesitate to seek help from a counsellor or your doctor if you're concerned. In cases of clinical depression, the doctor may recommend medication.

The mads are when you're so angry you're ready to blow. And because misery loves company, you want everyone else around you to be just as angry as you are. Need I say more?

The glads are when you get the giggles and you can't stop laughing. They're contagious, too. One person gets the glads and their hormones call to everyone else. Soon the whole class is laughing and no one knows why. This can be annoying for teachers in the classroom, or parents at the dinner table, but the glads are harmless overall.

When I'm teaching intermediates, I stress that the sads, mads and glads are normal and healthy during puberty, but it's important to find appropriate and respectful ways to deal with emotionally rough puberty days. Getting all "attitudey" with parents and teachers is not one of those ways. In the classroom, we brainstorm ideas that can help them cope without killing a sibling and getting themselves into deeper trouble. For example, maybe they need to have some down time in their room (self-imposed time outs can be invaluable). Or maybe they need to write in their journal to get their feelings out, or get in the bath and scream under water, or talk to a close friend or family member about what's bothering them. I'm always careful to mention that exercise is a great way to cope with the sads and mads. We know that exercise produces natural chemicals in the body called endorphins, which are scientifically proven to make us feel happy. I don't mean that they have to go run three miles, but even a brisk walk, a few times around the block can help.

A discussion of emotional changes at puberty wouldn't be complete without talking about crushes. It's totally normal for intermediates (and younger children as well) to develop romantic attraction to another person for the first time. It's also totally normal for intermediate children to not be the least bit interested in romance or relationships. When students bring up the topic in class, a common question from girls is, "If I think another girl is cute, does that mean I'm gay?" The answer is a simple "No." Adolescence is a time when children are figuring out who they are, and developing their sexual identity. The gender of the person who gives us butterflies in Grade 5, or even in Grade 11, doesn't necessarily indicate whether we are gay, straight, or something entirely different. Sometimes it does, but other times it doesn't.

Regardless, I think the most important thing for parents to remember when it comes to crushes is that they can be all consuming, intense, exhilarating, and embarrassing. Be open to talking with your child about their crushes, and take their feelings seriously. You may also want to remind your child that everyone has different comfort levels with crushes, and while they may feel totally comfortable with their crush being featured in morning announcements at school, for some people that would be horrifying. Respect for personal boundaries and privacy is super important here. It would also be great if you could share the ups and downs of your own childhood crushes with your intermediate child, to show that they are a real, fun, and harmless part of growing up.

> *Why did Mother Nature make growing up so hard? It is really frustrating!*

■ HOORAY FOR HEALTHY BODIES!

I find that kids at this age have a pretty good grasp of what healthy nutrition looks like. When talking about puberty with intermediates, though, I spend a few minutes stressing the importance of fuelling one's body with what it needs in order to grow and do the activities they want to do. I'm by no means a nutritionist, but I suggest the children use moderation in their eating. There's no food they can *never* have, but if they eat healthy stuff like veggies, protein, grains, dairy, and fruits 80% of the time, that leaves 20% for foods that may not be as healthy.

It's a no-brainer that kids should not be dieting, and I find that most parents are on top of that. But given that being gluten-free, dairy-free, sugar-free, etc. is trendy in our society right now, I encourage parents to make sure their children aren't limiting the foods they're eating without good reason.

We also need to remember that what we drink is part of our nutrition. I see way too many kids on the playground at recess with a giant bottle of Gatorade or other sports drink in their hand. Yes, these drinks can replace electrolytes in the body lost during profuse sweating, vomiting, and diarrhea. But no one needs them at school. Sport drinks should go in the "pop" category, consumed only once in a while. We also need to encourage kids (once they can read, of course) to check labels on their drinks. If it says "fruit *drink*," it's not juice. Look for added sugar and artificial flavouring too. Again, I'm not a nutritionist, but a glass of milk or milk substitute with dinner is a good idea, especially if kids aren't really into calcium-rich foods. Water is the healthiest drink of all. I love it when I go into a classroom and find water bottles on all of the desks. It's a good sign of a healthy class, and sipping water as we work is a great habit to start early!

For children aged five to 17, Canadian Physical Activity Guidelines suggest at least 60 minutes of moderate to vigorous-intensity physical

---

[Handwritten note: What is the best way to let out your anger]

activity at least three days a week, and 60 minutes of activities that strengthen muscle and bone at least three days a week. This doesn't mean training for a half marathon. Again, moderation is the key. Don't just talk about the health benefits of exercise, but about exercise for fun, stress release, socializing, teamwork, and energy burning as well. As I mentioned earlier, exercise also produces endorphins in the body, so it helps us to feel good emotionally. Insist that your children get some exercise every day, but don't ever force your child to do a sport or activity they hate. Most kids have plenty of activities to choose from, so do what you can to work with their interests.

BEYOND THE BOOGEYMAN

I tell children that scientists say that growth hormones are released in our bodies when we're fast asleep. This means that all young people (teenagers included) need extra sleep from time to time. In fact, every child needs a "heavy-duty-growing-night" at least once a week. I tell kids that when their parents are making dinner they can take one look at them and know right away if tonight is a heavy-duty-growing-night. Fighting with siblings, whining, complaining about the dinner, not doing chores or not turning off devices as soon as they're asked are all sure signs that they need sleep.

Adults sometimes need heavy-duty-growing-nights too, often in direct relation to the ages of their children. Like many adults today, you may have delayed your childbearing into your late 30s or 40s. You may have a blended family, and by the time you get both yours and your partner's children into puberty, you may be going through hormonal changes yourself. Some evenings the whole family is swinging from the chandeliers, which means everyone needs to go to bed early!

Seriously, though, some puberty-aged children can be plagued by sleep disturbances and be wide awake for hours after their normal bedtime. And some children, especially those who are going through an active growth spurt, have night terrors. These usually happen as they're trying to sleep and they're overcome with irrational fears. They can cry, shake, cling, feel nauseated, and be just plain terrified. "What if there is an earthquake, a tsunami, or some other natural disaster?" "What if you die, Mom or Dad, what would I do?" "What if I die?" "What if my dog dies, or what if I got a dog and then it died?" News stories, TV shows, and video games often trigger these fears, or a member of the child's extended family or community experiences a tragedy and sets them worrying.

I suggest that we always treat fears seriously and do some problem solving when it makes sense. Exactly what could they do in an emergency? Show your child the earthquake kits in place in your home. Make a list of emergency numbers and include any relatives or friends that you would trust with your children. Walk them through the escape plan they should use if there was a fire or a flood. Children feel huge relief when they feel empowered to handle an emergency. Assure them that you trust them and are confident that they can cope.

When it comes to normal sleep patterns, parents should recognize that all children don't necessarily need the same amount of sleep, just like adults. I do believe that children need a regular bedtime and that they should be in their beds (or at least in their bedroom) at the same time every night, with reasonable exceptions for weekends and special occasions, of course. But I also think that it could be unhealthy for them to be forced to lie in the dark for hours on end, unable to sleep. Maybe they could have a bedside light on and be allowed to read for a bit, do some writing, or listen to some calming music. No screens, of course, as we know that the light from screens reduces melatonin in the body making it even more difficult to get to sleep.

The bedtime routine can be especially challenging for a parent whose own sleep patterns are radically different from their child's. Try to be flexible and to allow children to discover, through puberty, their own best sleep patterns. That doesn't mean that we should allow our "night owl" children to be up roaming the house. Offer sleep aids – bedtime snacks, hot milk drinks, warm baths, hot water bottles, a back or foot rub, a bedtime story and relaxation time starting well before bedtime – but then insist that they stay in their beds.

■ MODELLING HEALTHY RELATIONSHIPS

Another common worry for intermediates that can cause sleep disturbances is "What if you and Mom (or Dad) get divorced?" What they are really asking is, "What will happen to me?" If you can, reassure them that a breakup is not on the agenda – *if you can*. Please don't lie to them if it's a real possibility. I know first-hand that marriage (or any long term relationship) is a lot of work. But if there's open verbal or physical abuse in your relationship, it's not surprising that your child is scared, worried, and sleepless.

Reassure your child that none of your relationship difficulties are their fault. Without giving too much information or venting like you would with a friend, be honest about how difficult relationships can be sometimes. You may need counselling (in fact, I think even the healthiest relationships get stronger with counselling) and if your partner won't go, go alone. Some therapists only see couples together and some want the whole family involved. I've found that a combination of the two can be valuable. But the bottom line is that children have the right to feel safe and secure in their home, and we need to provide that for our kids.

Putting children first can sometimes mean that a breakup is necessary. I'm not a therapist, but I know that there are toxic relationships that harm children, especially those that involve abuse of substances or power (especially when violence is used). Leave your partner if it means a healthier life for you and your children. When asked, sometimes children want their parents to separate, and they are willing to accept a lower standard of living, or a single parent situation, in order to have some peace, security, and consistency in their lives. They also want both their parents to be happy. Putting children first doesn't mean that they rule the household or have complete control. But your relationship decisions will inform their own relationships someday. Model maturity for them, and don't settle for anything less than a healthy relationship.

■ WEIGHT GAIN AND BODY IMAGE

Remember that the weight children need to gain during puberty usually happens over ten years, but kids in puberty gain weight in different ways. Some kids gain their puberty weight really quickly in elementary school, before they get taller, so they may feel self-conscious because they're chubbier than their friends. Other kids gain their puberty weight very gradually throughout elementary and high school as they get taller, so they feel self-conscious because they're skinner or lankier than their friends. Regardless, our kids need to know that gaining weight as they grow up is necessary and normal.

But it's not as simple as that. Despite that parents often use every chance they get to reassure their children that their bodies are perfect just as they are, kids today are struggling with poor body image at record young ages. The Canadian Women's Foundation reports that 50% of Grade 6 girls have been on a diet. Not surprisingly, dissatisfaction with one's body can lead to struggles with self-esteem, disordered eating, and self-harm. Indeed, MediaSmarts reports that in a national U.S. study in 2008, 25% of girls who identified as having low self-esteem also reported disordered eating (compared to 7% of girls with high self-esteem), and 25% of girls with low self-esteem injured themselves on purpose (compared to 4% of girls with high self-esteem). The Canadian Women's Foundation also tells us that 50% of girls wish they were someone else, and that nine out of ten feel pressure from the media to be thin. This is serious stuff.

Parents often tell me that they've had repeated discussions with their children stressing that being healthy and strong is much more important than how their body looks. They also have gone on endlessly about how a person's appearance doesn't help them achieve their major goals in life. The old "What matters is on the inside" speech does have some value as filler in a broader context (especially if it's coming from someone other than a parent), but still, our children are struggling.

For girls, it's about playing a comparison game with unrealistically thin models in magazines, wannabe YouTube stars, and whoever they

FUN FACT: Children need to gain about 35 pounds during puberty in order to be healthy.

follow on Instagram. It's a game that's impossible to win, and some lingerie retailers – whose ads tell them they need to look sexy at age 14 – don't help either. (How those companies sexualize preteens makes me sick, but I won't get started on that.)

I want to make it clear, though, that poor body image isn't just a problem for girls. Eating disorders are also on the rise among boys, particularly athletes (*Reuters*, January 8, 2009). There are also concerns that some boys – some as young as age 10 – are becoming obsessed with building a muscular physique (National Strength and Conditioning Association, June 3, 2009).

Boys also get strong messages early in life about what it means to be attractive or sexy. Take Batman, for example. In the 1960s, this beloved superhero used to have a bit of a belly and look quite soft under his grey or blue spandex unitard. Today, Batman is 200 pounds of solid muscle dressed head to toe in armour. Musicians and actors that boys look up to, even young ones, have 12-pack abs, not to mention a very obvious lack of body hair. To make matters worse, modern gender stereotypes teach boys that they should have good bodies, but not show that they care or try too hard. Their looks should be effortless; obsessing about bodies should be left to girls and gay guys.

> *Are the girls in our class overweight or underweight*

So how can we help our children rise above this pressure? This is a tough one and even I feel hopeless some days. But here are some ideas, tactics I've found helpful over the years when it comes to my own girls:

1. Never, ever say any of these things to your child.

"Do you really need another piece of bread before your dinner comes?"
"You're not fat, just bigger boned than your sister."
"Why don't we try to lose a few pounds together?"
"Doing cross country this term will help you lose some of that baby fat."
"When you reach your goal weight, I'll buy you those jeans you've been wanting."

These comments are demeaning and only reinforce our society's obsession with weight.

2. Check yourself. How do you feel about your own body?

Are you obsessed with losing weight? Try not to trash your body in front of the mirror when your child is around. And don't say things like, "I'm not eating carbs," or "I gotta lose my beer belly before summer!" Children internalize the negativity. Don't diet, and don't be afraid to give yourself compliments. For example, over dinner some night, you could share, **"I had a great yoga class today. I'm so much more flexible than I was when I started going. I can tell that my hard work is paying off."**

3. Don't make comments, positive or negative, about your child's *body*.

If you'd like to comment about your child's *appearance*, say, **"You look so healthy,"** or **"You looked really strong at ballet today,"** or **"I love the outfit you chose today; you've always had great style."** If you think your daughter's body looks perfect in her new swimsuit, keep it to yourself. Instead, give compliments based only on personality characteristics, talents, and special qualities. For real.

4. Redefine beautiful. Beauty is not rail thin or super cut; it's strong and healthy and confident.

Celebrate authentic natural beauty. Images in fashion and sports magazines aren't real, so it's a waste of time to compare ourselves to them. Not only that, but research has shown us for years now that self-esteem plummets after reading a beauty or fashion magazine for even 10 minutes…at every age.

5. Use natural opportunities to teach about the reality of Hollywood.

For example, while watching the Oscars together, you could say, **"I wonder how these women would look tonight if they hadn't spent hours with the help of makeup artists, hair stylists, and wardrobe people?"**

6. Teach your child to be media literate.

Change the question from "What's wrong with my body?" to "What's wrong with this picture?" Think critically and ask questions like, **"Do cosmetics companies want us to feel good about how we look?"** Ask, **"Why do retailers market push-up bras to preteens?"** Pay attention to how men and women are portrayed in TV and film. Ask, **"Have you ever noticed that heroines in movies are usually thin and beautiful (by media standards) and evil female characters are often ugly and fat?"** Discuss song lyrics and the messages they send (more on that in a bit).

7. Encourage your child to make good choices about the media they consume.

Set reasonable limits and boundaries around what they watch, but let them know that you trust them to make good decisions even when you aren't around. As challenging as it can be, find TV shows and movies that reinforce your family values and beliefs. For my family, watching *Modern Family* together has been really great that way.

8. Teach your child that sports and other activities help us become healthier and stronger.

They also help us be better leaders, relieve stress, learn teamwork, and be more confident. Never force them to do an extracurricular activity they hate, and invite them to join you in exercise that you enjoy. Remind them that marathon runners come in all shapes and sizes, and that Olympic athletes don't have bodies like models. You can show your appreciation for this by making comments like, **"I find it so inspiring to watch women play hockey. They're so strong and powerful...now that's beautiful!"**

9. Model and teach balanced eating early on.

Have salad with pizza. Have a burger and fries once in a while and don't apologize for it or even comment on it. It's not always easy, but whenever possible carve out time to make dinner rather than grabbing something that can be put in the microwave. Kids can help prepare meals even before you get home from work. Sit down at the table for meals rather than eating in front of the TV or computer. The sooner these healthy habits are passed on to our children, the more likely they'll stick as they grow up and gain independence.

10. Teach your child that they're so much more than their physical body.

Empower them to stand up for what they believe in, even if it's not trendy. Celebrate the unique individuals they are at every opportunity. Recognize their kindness and other special qualities. Encourage them to do things they love, that challenge themselves and that help others.

■ WE'RE STILL BATTLING BULLYING

There's no shortage of resources for parents on helping children cope with bullying, so I'll only address it briefly here. Sadly, kids are being bullied at every age. But during the intermediate stage of development, when preteens are already so unsure of themselves as their body changes, bullying can be especially devastating. I want to be clear that bullying, whether it's physical, verbal, social, emotional (or whatever other label you'd like to attach to it) is *not* okay. No child needs to experience it as a "rite of passage" or as "part of growing up." There are simply too many young people being terrorized at school and in their communities and it needs to stop.

I know many of you are thinking, "Well that's a no brainer, Saleema!" And for most of us it is. I'm so happy and relieved to report that we've come a long way since we parents were growing up. Communities, schools, and even celebrities are now responding seriously to violence, bullying, and other unacceptable behaviour. Through initiatives such as the It Gets Better Project, Amanda Todd Legacy, and Pink Shirt Day (to name three of many), we've also come a long way in terms of teaching young people to come together as a society against bullying and harassment. We've put some responsibility, and rightfully so, on the bystander to take a stand in order to make someone else's situation a bit better.

We as adults need to listen to our children, help them to feel empowered, and teach them how to effectively deal with bullying. That is, we need to teach our kids how to be assertive. Assertiveness skills can be taught and used at any age and are invaluable in a variety of situations.

If your child comes to you with a bullying situation, help them understand that friendship and peer issues are unfortunately an inevitable part of life. Try not to rush into problem-solving mode, but be an empathetic listener. Your child needs you to understand that they're hurting and this is a big deal. More than advice, our kids want to feel validated. Help them identify feelings around the issue, and remind

> *Why would people have homophobia? I mean, everyone's encouraged to "be themselves," so this is so hypocritical.*

them that it is okay to feel angry, sad, and frustrated. Get the details about the situation and ask lots of open-ended questions: "How did the bullying start?" "How did you respond?" "What specifically upsets you most about the situation?"

Once you have a clear idea of what exactly happened and how your child is feeling, then ask them what they think would be the best way to solve the problem. As you are brainstorming ideas, teach or review the five steps to being assertive:

1. Use eye contact:
Looking at someone in the eyes conveys that you mean what you say. If you're too uncomfortable, look between their eyes or at their eyebrows – they won't be able to tell.

2. Have a strong body:
Non-verbal communication is even more powerful than our words, so make sure your physical body reflects confidence. Plant your feet firmly on the ground and keep your hands at your side. Keep your chin up and shoulders back. Avoid fidgeting, it shows nervousness.

3. Use an "I" statement:

Tell the person how their behaviour makes you feel. For example, you could say, "I don't like it when you call me names," or "I want you to stop harassing me," or "I feel sad when you talk about me behind my back." The great thing about I statements is that no one can argue with your feelings, and it's tough to think of a smart comeback! If they do respond, repeat the I statement, but no more than two times. Remember that bullies want a reaction from their victims, it gives them power. If we have a calm, assertive response and don't engage them, we keep our power. At iGirl, our empowerment workshop for girls aged 9–12, facilitator Ashley McIntosh explains it best when she teaches participants that the key is to be "boring to bully."

4. Have a strong voice:

Don't yell, but be firm.

5. Walk away and report:

Don't run; it can be interpreted as fear. And if your assertiveness skills don't seem to be working, get the help of an adult.

Understandably, many children are hesitant to tell an adult what's going on for fear that this will aggravate the bully and make things worse. They also don't want to be labelled as a tattletale. But we need to teach our kids the difference between *ratting* and *reporting*. I explain it to kids this way: "**Ratting is telling on someone for the sole purpose of getting them into trouble (e.g., rushing to tell the teacher when you see Jamie writing on their desk). Reporting, on the other hand, is telling on someone to keep yourself or someone else *out* of trouble. Especially if you have used your best assertiveness skills over and over again, but the situation isn't getting any better, you need to report.**" The "or someone else" part is super important here. We have huge power to help others by reporting, especially when they don't have assertiveness skills or the confidence to report for themselves.

Being a responsible bystander and standing up for others is crucial. If we don't say or do anything, we send the message that the behaviour is okay, or that we don't care. Don't be afraid to ask your school how they're making the situation better for your child. Administration and staff have a responsibility to provide a safe learning environment for all children.

As useful as assertiveness may be in real-life bullying situations, we need different strategies to deal with cyberbullying. I'll talk specifically about that in the next chapter.

RESOURCES

FOR PARENTS

WEBSITES
- www.participaction.com
- www.mediasmarts.ca
- www.amandatoddlegacy.org
- www.pinkshirtday.ca
- www.itgetsbetter.org
- www.sexualityandu.ca
- www.teachingsexualhealth.ca
- www.kidshealth.org
- www.iwannaknow.org
- www.sexplainer.com
- www.lunapads.com
- www.gday.world (G Day is a global social movement with events across Canada celebrating girls' transition to adolescence.)

BOOKS
- *Masterminds and Wingmen: Helping Our Boys Cope with Schoolyard Power, Locker-Room Tests, Girlfriends, and the New Rules of Boy World,* by Rosalind Wiseman.
- *Odd Girl Out: Revised and Updated: The Hidden Culture of Aggression in Girls,* by Rachel Simmons.
- *Queen Bees and Wannabes: Helping Your Daughter Survive Cliques, Gossip, Boyfriends, and the New Realities of Girl World*, by Rosalind Wiseman.

ARTICLES
- *How to Talk to Your Daughter about Her Body,* by Sarah Koppelkam. http://www.huffingtonpost.com/sarah-koppelkam/body-image_b_3678534.html

FOR INTERMEDIATE CHILDREN

WEBSITES AND YOUTUBE CLIPS

- *Camp Gyno*, a hilarious ad about getting a period at camp. https://www.youtube.com/watch?v=0XnzfRqkRxU
- *First Moon Party*, another hilarious ad about a girl faking her first period and paying the price. https://www.youtube.com/watch?v=NEcZmT0fiNM. Both by www.helloflo.com.
- www.beinggirl.com
- www.boyslife.com
- www.amysmartgirls.com (Founded by artist Amy Poehler, this organization is dedicated to helping young people cultivate their authentic selves.)

BOOKS

- *All Made Up: A Girl's Guide to Seeing through Celebrity Hype and Celebrating Real Beauty,* by Audrey D. Brashich.
- *Am I Weird or Is This Normal?* by Marlin S. Potash and Laura Potash Fruitman.
- *Happier Periods Naturally: The G Day Guide to Natural Periods,* a booklet by Madeleine Shaw and Suzanne Siemens, founders of Lunapads International Products Ltd, Vancouver, BC. www.lunapads.com.
- *It's Amazing!,* by Robie H. Harris.
- *It's Perfectly Normal: Changing Bodies, Growing Up, and Sexual Health,* by Robie H. Harris.
- *My Body, Myself for Boys/My Body, Myself for Girls*, by Lynda and Area Madaras.
- *Puberty Boy,* by Geoff Price.
- *Puberty Girl*, by Shushann Movsessian.
- *Stick Up for Yourself! Every Kid's Guide to Personal Power and Positive Self-Esteem,* by L. Raphael and G. Kaufman.
- *The Body Book for Boys,* by Grace Norwich.
- *The Boy's Body Book: Everything You Need to Know for Growing Up You,* by Kelli Dunham.

- *The Care and Keeping of You and other American Girl Series* for girls aged 8 and up. (These books offer valuable support and guidance on a range of emotional and academic issues associated with growing up.)
- *The Looks Book: A Whole New Approach to Beauty, Body Image, and Style* by the creators of www.gurl.com.
- *What's Happening to Me?,* by Peter Mayle.
- *What's Happening to Me?,* by Usborne Books www.usborne.com. (One book for boys, one book for girls.)

MAGAZINES
- *American Girl*, ages 7 and up www.americangirl.com
- *Discovery Girls*, ages 8 and up www.discoverygirls.com
- *New Moon*, ages 8 and up, www.newmoon.org
- *Vervegirl*, ages 13 and up, www.vervegirl.com

6. Managing Media and the Internet

6. Managing Media and the Internet

■ INTERMEDIATES (GRADES 4 AND 5)

No one would argue that over the last decade the Internet has dramatically changed the way we consume media and interact with others. Indeed, in their 2015 YCWW Phase III study, MediaSmarts reports that in 2004, only 36% of Canadians were even connected to the Internet. There was no Facebook, Skype, or YouTube, and the first Blackberry was still years away. Today, one quarter of students in Grade 4 have their own smart phones. The numbers increase steadily until phone ownership hits 85% in Grade 11.

MediaSmarts also reports that one third of students in Grades 4 to 6 have Facebook accounts even though the website's terms of use prohibit anyone under the age of 13 from joining. YouTube is the single most popular site across all age groups (with the exception of girls in Grades 7 to 11, who placed it second after Facebook) and, for the first time, young people are getting more of their media from the Internet than from television.

The explosion of social media sites has also made it easier for preteens and teens to create an online presence or persona. Three quarters now have a social media profile or blog, which is a 250% increase over the number of students who had personal sites in 2005.

Given these dramatic changes, there's no doubt that the Internet has changed our lives in a major way at every age. On the plus side, it's never been easier to connect with others over long distances, collect information, learn, shop, work, play games, and access entertainment.

TALK SEX TODAY

FUN FACT:
I got my first cell phone when I was **26 years** old.

What this means, though, is that we parents need to support and guide our children through their digital world – a world that's drastically different than the one we grew up in.

Understandably, this stresses parents out. Particularly for intermediate children, the Internet can have a profound influence on how they develop and discover their identity. Nine- and ten-year-olds are learning how to "look hot at a party" from YouTube tutorials. They're comparing themselves to posts of friends and even strangers online, and are watching sexually graphic (and often misogynistic) music videos. They're playing violent online games with people they don't know, can access pornography with the push of a button, and are sleeping with their phones for fear they'll miss a message from a friend. At the same time, as intermediates naturally gain more freedom, get smart phones, and spend more time away from home, monitoring their online activity becomes increasingly difficult for parents.

How, then, do we make sure our kids stay safe online? How do we stay involved in their social lives when so much of their interaction with their friends happens on a device? How do we protect them from the misinformation and sexually explicit content they might find online? How do we protect their privacy? And what about all the horror stories we hear about sexting, cyberbullying, and predators? With so much at stake, it's not surprising that parents are losing sleep.

Before you think I'm a total Debbie Downer, let's talk about the good news. Yes, the fact that our children live in a digital world can be problematic and the issues related to this need to be dealt with. But we also need to remember that, for the large majority of our youth, being online is a positive experience. If we set that reality as our frame of reference, it allows us to take on this aspect of parenting calmly, rather than with panic or paranoia. From this calm place, we need to focus our energy on teaching our children responsible decision-making online, especially when we're not around. We also need to show them how to be respectful digital citizens, and clearly communicate our expectations for online behaviour. Equally important, parents should assure their children that they can come to them for help when needed. If we do this earlier rather than later, good online habits will be formed long before the teen years. And let's face it – a little push back in the intermediate years is better than all-out war when our kids are 15!

So where do we begin? While I respect that different styles work for different families, I take a pretty hard-line approach to children being online. For starters, long before our kids get a smart phone in their hands, they need to understand that having a device and using the Internet is a *privilege*, not a *right*. We all have to act responsibly, maturely and ethically online. If children don't, this privilege should get taken away. I think many parents find it difficult to enforce rules around the Internet (and lots of other things) because they don't want their children to be mad at them. *But our job as parents is not to be our child's friend.* Let me say it again: *Our job as parents is not to be our child's friend.* If our kids get mad at us when we follow through with rules and boundaries, it means we're doing something right!

I'm not claiming for one second that I know all the answers when it comes to keeping our kids safe and happy online, but I'd like to offer some general suggestions based on what I know about kids' digital lives. Many of these have worked well in my home over the years.

Embrace the Internet. As foreign as it may be to you, bring yourself up to speed on how children interact online. Get comfortable with texting and texting abbreviations. Text your kids. Be familiar with the social media websites and apps they're using. Post every now and then.

Talk to your child about how critical thinking and smart decision-making will make being online a really positive experience for them. This means, **"Don't believe everything you see or read online and don't participate in behaviour that's mean."**

Make sure your kids know you trust them to use good judgment. You could say, **"I'm so proud of the good decisions you've made in lots of areas of your life, and I know you'll do that online as well. If you ever run into trouble though, I'm here to support you."** Children need to feel that their parents trust them. It gives them confidence and also puts a little pressure on them to prove their parents right.

Keep screens out of bedrooms. Instead, put all TVs and computers in "public" areas of your home.

Set limits on screen time (the number of hours per day, as well as appropriate times, for example, not at the dinner table) and determine when devices should be in a central charging station at night (that includes yours!).

Communicate to your child that there's no privacy online because the Internet is a public space. As children learn the ins and outs of the digital world, parents have a responsibility to monitor their children's activity and need to know their passwords at all times. *This isn't about control or power, it's about safety.* A parent could explain this by saying, **"I trust that you make smart decisions online, which is why I'm not going to monitor your every post. But from time to time, because your safety is my responsibility, I may need to access your accounts and activity. My hope is that we can do this together, but it may need to be without your knowledge. I'm confident, though, that this won't be an issue for us."**

Be assertive and make decisions that work for your family. For example, don't get your child a cell phone just because all their friends have one... and delay this for as long as possible! Personally, I can't see a child needing a cell phone before high school, unless they're travelling on public transit to and from elementary school.

Now let's talk about the more specific aspects of your intermediate child's online life.

■ TV, MOVIES, AND YOUTUBE CLIPS

At my house, it's rare that my stepdaughters sit down to watch a movie or TV show in front of our flat screen in the living room. Instead, they're on their laptops with earbuds in. I can be in the same room and have no idea what they are watching unless I hover over their shoulder, which I sometimes do. This is less of an issue with teens, but for parents with intermediates who are more easily influenced by what they're exposed to in media, it's concerning. How can we moderate the influence of media when we don't even know what they're watching? Trust, lots of talking, and clear expectations and boundaries are steps in the right direction.

Decide together which TV shows, movies, and YouTube clips are age-appropriate. If you're unsure about a specific TV show your child is asking to watch, watch it together and then make a decision. We can learn much from our child's reaction to and interest in certain shows and an added bonus is the opportunity to talk. Don't be afraid to rule out content that's sexually graphic or violent. You could say, **"We're not okay with you watching adult-rated TV shows and movies at your age. Not only are they inappropriate, but you don't yet have the life experience to really understand and make sense of what you are seeing and hearing. As you get older you'll have more freedom to watch shows with more adult content."**

Remember that *appropriateness* is different from *personal taste*. You may question why on earth your child would want to waste time watching a 20-minute YouTube tutorial on how to braid hair a certain way, but don't judge or criticize. Express your preference for the more interesting, useful, or entertaining clips they choose to watch. Share some of your favourites.

[handwritten: Why is sex mentioned on TV so much lately?]

Discuss how so-called "reality" shows aren't real at all. Shows about teenage pregnancy, for example, glamourize and trivialize the challenges faced by a teen parent. They portray romance between young parents, and a new found maturity and independence that don't usually exist in real life.

Even if shows don't claim to be reality shows, question storylines and whether their outcomes would happen in real life. **"Do you think someone would get away with using that level of violence in real life? What would be the consequences?"**

Discuss how popular TV shows aimed at youth don't represent the typical life of a preteen or teen. Based on what intermediates see on these shows, it's easy to believe that all teens are having sex five times a week, either in relationships or by just hooking up. Not true.

Draw your child's attention to gender stereotypes and how women are represented in media. **"In real life, do you think men are always** more focused on their careers than women are?" "How do relationships in movies compare with the relationships you see in real life?"

Don't forget marketing. **"Who are cosmetics companies marketing to?" "Do they want people to feel good about themselves?" "What would happen if people decided they liked how they look without these products?"**

■ ONLINE GAMING

Although the findings are inconsistent, much of the research tells us that too much exposure to online games raises aggression and lowers empathy in children. While we need to recognize that violent video games affect every child differently, parents can intervene. I'm by no means an authority on online gaming (although I do play a mean game of solitaire on my iPad) but here are some tips from the experts Common Sense Media and MediaSmarts. As you read, keep in mind that when kids play online games they develop relationships with the people they're playing with – kind of like in a chatroom. Most of these people are harmless, but some could put your child at risk.

Just like it's important to know what our kids are watching on TV, we need to be familiar with the games they're playing online.

Whenever possible, join your children while they play games, even if it's just watching. Not only is it interesting to see what type of games they are attracted to, but this allows for a covert risk assessment. Maybe it's not as bad as you think!

Use ratings for guidance but don't rely solely on them because they're often given by players and are, therefore, subjective.

Read the "Terms and Conditions," "Game Policies," or "Parents" section of each game to see whether or not chat is moderated, how to report inappropriate conduct, how to block harassing players, if personal information is collected, and if so, how it is used.

Come to an agreement with your child in terms of how much of their time should be spent gaming, and how they will make sure that gaming doesn't interfere with other activities and responsibilities in their life. Check to see if any of the games your child is interested in playing has a minimum weekly number of hours of play before registering or progressing to higher levels.

Talk about the potential impact violence and sexually graphic content in gaming can have, especially when games glorify violence or demean women.

Find ways to say "yes." Look on reputable websites such as www.commonsensemedia.org for reviews of online games, and encourage your child to choose games that have educational value or that encourage social responsibility and leadership skills rather than consumerism.

Be true to yourself. Different aspects of games are more important to some than others, so stay in your comfort zone. If coarse language or violence really get to you, don't be afraid to place those games in the "no-go" category for your child.

Check yourself. Model healthy gaming habits and walk the talk!

PREDATORS

In Grades 4 and 5, online gaming is one of the easiest ways for predators to gain access to children. Even on seemingly harmless websites like Club Penguin, children (without even realizing it) can give private information to people they're playing with thinking they're kids their age. And, if a child is having a tough time at school or is being bullied by other players on the site, they're vulnerable to being lured into meeting someone who wants to be their "friend" in person.

Of course, this isn't always the case. Most people in the world are kind, safe, and caring. But we need to preload our children with the skills they need to keep themselves safe in the real world *and* online. We don't want to instill paranoia in our kids unnecessarily, but they need to know that there are people online who pretend to be someone they're not, or who try to bribe children with compliments or money. Because we know this, we need to be really mindful about who

> *What does "predators" mean?*

we let into our lives, who we share personal information with, and who we trust. Even the smartest people can give away personal information online without realizing it. For example, someone could post a team photo after their soccer game. Now a predator can use the jerseys to pinpoint where exactly their team practices. Predators can also use the background of a photo to figure out its location. Later in this chapter, I'll suggest some specific Internet rules that can help your child stay safe from predators.

■ MUSIC

From day one, music is such an important part of our lives. I have great memories of listening to the Top 40 countdown on the radio on Saturday mornings in elementary and high school, desperately trying to press play record on the tape recorder at exactly the right time when the Top 10 songs came on. Admittedly, my favourites (including Madonna's "Like a Virgin" and "Papa Don't Preach," a song about teenage pregnancy) were pretty racy at the time, but they didn't even come close to the suggestive, sexual and misogynistic nature of pop and rap music today. Plus, it wasn't in our faces as much. The only time we could watch music videos, for example, was on the TV show *Friday Night Videos*. Today, our Grade 4 and 5 kids can watch videos for free on YouTube as many times as they like. And wow, they sure are different from 30 years ago.

And then there are the lyrics. I'm not saying that sexually graphic, misogynistic lyrics didn't exist when we were growing up, of course they did. But I would argue they've been taken up a few notches. An example that first comes to mind is Bruno Mars' song "Gorilla." I couldn't believe my eyes when I read the lyrics online recently (Google "Gorilla lyrics"). Glamourizing casual sex, using offensive language, normalizing sexual violence, promoting the subordination and degradation of a woman… I've enjoyed this singer for years as a fun, unique, respectful, kid-friendly artist, but this song infuriated me. Talk about reinforcing rape culture and the gender stereotypes we're so desperately trying to get rid of!

But can we stop our kids from listening to the radio? No. Can we control every song they hear? No, especially as they get older. And should we ban them from listening to Bruno Mars ever again? Of course not. What we *can* do, though, is have meaningful conversations about song lyrics and the messages they send to listeners. These conversations can start long before the intermediate years.

I remember a time a few years ago when the topic of song lyrics came up in a Grade 1 class I was teaching. We had just finished talking about reproduction through sexual intercourse and, as I often do, I asked the class, "Have you heard of sex before?" A chorus of students exclaimed, "Yah!" One of the students specified that he had heard of it "because there is a song on the radio that says, 'Hey, sexy lady!'" Another six-year-old added, "And there's also a song that says, 'I'm sexy and I know it!'"

Loving this unexpected teachable moment, I responded, "That's right, and I'm so glad this came up. Now that you've learned that sex is only for grown-ups, do you think it would be appropriate for kids to sing those songs or even use the word 'sexy'?" Being the rule followers they are at this age, the whole class responded, "No way! That would be *so* inappropriate!" We did a quick brainstorm of more appropriate terms they could substitute for the word "sexy" in a song. "Hey, *funny* lady," "Hey, *smart* lady," "I'm *happy* and I know it." Then one of the girls said, "Yah, but you know what, Saleema? Some kids say things that are way more inappropriate than 'sexy.' Like this one boy in Grade 6, you know what he says? (a hush comes over the crowd) He says 'pathetic.'" Her appalled classmates gasped, unable to accept that someone in their school would use such profanity.

Yes, talking to littles about music lyrics is relatively easy and fun because they appreciate boundaries and rules to help regulate their own as well as their peers' behaviour. But how can a parent deal with a preteen who claims the parent is just being controlling, totally uncool, and are overreacting to music "everyone listens to" and that doesn't affect them in a negative way? There's no simple answer, but what I found helpful when my stepdaughters were younger was to discuss in detail why I was uncomfortable with them listening to a specific song or artist.

One time when Afton and Kate were eight and ten, we were driving with my mother-in-law who was visiting for the weekend. We were listening to the radio and the girls freaked out when Lady Gaga's song featuring the lyrics "I wanna take a ride on your disco stick" came on and I changed the station. In an effort to practice what I preach, I pulled over, hoping that my mother-in-law wouldn't be forever traumatized by the conversation I was about to have with her granddaughters. Long story short, both girls were shocked to learn that the "disco stick" being referred to in the song was a penis.

Even more puzzling to them was that someone would sing about something so personal, and they claimed that they no longer liked the song. Did they swear off Lady Gaga forever? Not at all. All three of us appreciate her as a gifted artist. But more importantly, they left the conversation (I hope) with more understanding, and a realization of the fact that song lyrics can be very sexual without seeming to be so. I challenged them to listen to songs more critically, and stressed that they could always come to me if they had questions or concerns about what they were listening to.

That specific conversation went as well as I could have hoped. Stepmom of the year, right? Even my mother-in-law handled it like a pro. But, since then, we have had many more challenging exchanges about music. One of these conversations centred around a rapper I find extremely misogynistic (not to mention violent and sexually explicit) in his lyrics and general attitude. Afton and Kate battled with me over the fact that I wouldn't allow them to download any music by him. They swore up and down that they disagreed with what he was singing and didn't pay attention to the words, but argued that they still had the right make their own decisions about the music they enjoyed. They had a point, but I held my ground and explained my concern. It went something like this.

"I know that music is really important to you and that it plays a big role in how you express yourself. I support that 100%, and I'm not trying to control which artists or types of music you like. But I *do* think you are old enough and smart enough to think carefully about what you choose to listen to. When you purchase or even listen to music that's disrespectful, degrading, or violent towards women, you're

indirectly supporting those attitudes. This music is not only age inappropriate for you, I don't think it's appropriate for people of *any* age. When it comes to songs that are sexually explicit, or that downplay the seriousness and specialness of a sexual relationship, I worry that they'll influence your attitudes and maybe even your behaviour in one way or another. Do you understand where I'm coming from? What do you think?"

The more conversations like this we have with our preteens and teens, the more our message will stick. The hope is that eventually they'll make ethical choices about the music they listen to or, at the very least, question the message. Equally important as having these tricky conversations is to wholeheartedly support our kids in their love for artists who are positive role models for young people. Spring for a family Spotify subscription, give concert tickets as birthday presents, and rock out to music that's appropriate for people of all ages to listen to. Come on, who doesn't love a good karaoke session on the way to swim practice?

■ SOCIAL MEDIA

Thanks to social media, the world is smaller than ever. Facebook, Instagram, and other sites have allowed us to share and socialize with others in a way that we never have before. In fact, starting in the intermediate years, much of our kids' interactions with their peers happens on social media. This also gives parents a chance to connect with their children and teens in a way that our parents never could. I have to admit – it always feels good when one of my stepdaughters "likes" a photo or an article I've posted. And when they post photos while away at school, it sure makes them feel not so far away.

But social media also allows our kids to exist and interact in a world we know relatively little about and can easily be kept from us. (Parents, let's not be too hard on ourselves; we didn't have the Internet growing up.) What's more, how a young person behaves and represents themselves on social media can have a huge impact on them, not only today, but years down the road.

For this reason, I urge parents to develop rules, limits, and guidelines early on specifically around their child's social media activity. Not all parents will agree with me, but I tend to take a more hands-on approach when it comes to our responsibility (and right) to monitor all aspects of our children's social media activity. Again, this becomes more challenging as children move into the teen years, but here are some basic suggestions for discussing what's appropriate for "entry-level" social media users.

Be your child's friend/follower on social media. Post every now and then. Have a presence in their online life.

Talk to your child about Facebook, Instagram, Snapchat, and other

---

HERE'S AN EXAMPLE OF SOME SOCIAL MEDIA RULES WE TEACH IN OUR iGIRL EMPOWERMENT WORKSHOPS FOR GIRLS:

Granny Rule

DON'T send or post anything to anyone you wouldn't feel comfortable with the whole world seeing, including your Granny.
DO remember that the Internet is public – private comments or photos don't belong.
DO remember that your body is the most important, special, private thing you own…Granny would agree!

Toothbrush Rule

DO treat your passwords like your toothbrush: change them regularly and don't share them with anyone (except your parents).

Creep Rule

DON'T do anything someone you've met online asks you to do, especially when you know it's something your parents wouldn't be happy about.
DO choose a safe screen name for yourself that won't reveal personal information about you or your family.
DON'T share your personal information online or with someone you meet online. This includes your name, address, phone number, age, school name, passport number, or bank information.
DO make your personal safety your priority, knowing that there are some people online who pretend to be someone they're not, or who may try to bribe you with compliments or money.
DON'T call or agree to get together with anyone you've "met" online without

social networking apps specifically about
- the risk of creating a public persona that may not reflect who they really are
- the impact of others making judgments about their character based on what they see in social media
- the danger of fuelling their self-esteem with likes and comments
- the negative consequences of spending hours "connecting" with people on social media when they could be connecting with friends in real life
- "Facebook envy," the damaging effects of comparing one's real life with the best 10% of others

checking with a parent first, or without a parent coming with you.

PG (Parental Guidance) Rule

DO tell your parents if you come across anything online that makes you feel uncomfortable or scared, such as photos, videos, links to adult web sites, or messages with disrespectful language.

DON'T answer any emails or instant messages from people you don't know, or from anyone your parents have not approved.

DON'T send anything to someone you've met online without checking with your parents first.

DO check with a parent before sending someone your photo online.

DON'T send hurtful messages online and, if you receive one, don't respond to it or forward it. Instead, print it and report it to your parents.

DO respect your parents' house rules and limits for the Internet (for example, "No devices in the bedroom"). Those rules are there because your parents love you and want to keep you safe.

DO share with your parents some of your favourite things to do online so you can have fun together and learn cool new stuff.

Think Rule

DO make sure that what you are posting is **T**rue, **H**onest, **I**ntelligent (and **I**nteresting), **N**ecessary, and **K**ind.

DO treat others the way you would like to be treated. Use good manners when online, including respectful language and only kind words.

Ask your child questions to help them make their own decisions about how they want to spend their time. **"What's important to you each day?" "Which activities make your heart sing?" "How does reading people's Facebook posts make you feel?" "Do you think people post all aspects of their lives on social media, or only the good stuff?"**

Rally the troops. Ask friends and family to help send these positive messages to your child about social media. Recruit parents of your child's friends to present a united front (for example, Sarah's mom and I have decided that we aren't comfortable with you girls using ask.fm). Invite speakers to visit your school to reinforce what you've taught in a slightly different way. Hearing it from the "expert" is very powerful. Discuss stories in the media and cut out newspaper articles that will help you have a general discussion about why the principles you're teaching are so important. Life-saving, actually. Sadly, there are countless tragedies to refer to.

> what do you do when you get caught in an online sexual relationship that you don't feel comfortable with?

Use the above suggestions to develop a list of social media rules for your family. Explain to your child that, as they get older, they'll have more freedom in terms of what they consume and when, as well as in terms of how involved you are in monitoring their activity. But stress that, even when they're outside your home, you expect them to follow these rules. If not, then you'll need to monitor their use more closely and maybe even take their Internet privileges away.

■ BE HYPERAWARE OF HYPERSEXUALIZATION

Before we continue this discussion of managing media and see how it pertains to Grade 6 and 7 kids in the next chapter, we need to acknowledge that all the forms of media outlined above (and pop culture in general) contribute to the hypersexualization of youth, particularly girls, at younger and younger ages. In fact, according to Dr.

Blye Frank from the University of Dalhousie, "The challenges that a 14-year-old girl faced 20 years ago are the challenges faced by nine-year-old girls today." Sounds about right to me.

The Canadian Women's Health Network defines hyper-sexualization (also known as sexualization) as "girls being depicted or treated as sexual objects, with sexuality being inappropriately imposed on girls through media, marketing or products directed at them that encourage them to act in adult sexual ways." There are endless examples of hypersexualization in our society: "first date bras" being pushed on preteens, seven-year-olds wearing T-shirts that say "Flirt," YouTube tutorials teaching girls how to "get the guy you like to kiss you," and music videos featuring lingerie-clad women dancing provocatively around disinterested men wearing jeans and T-shirts, to name a few. Not to mention a "plastic surgery" mobile app encouraging children to perform cosmetic surgery on a virtual girl to make her "slim and beautiful." (After thousands of consumer complaints, the app was removed from Apple's App Store.)

Why do girls get so pressured to look a certain way?

Research by the American Psychological Association (APA) shows that seeing sexualized images of women causes many girls to be highly critical of their bodies, undermining their confidence and increasing feelings of shame, anxiety, and self-disgust. The APA has also found that hypersexualization impairs girls' ability to concentrate and links it to lowered physical activity, disordered eating, low self-esteem, and depression. Hypersexualization (and the resulting self-objectification) has also been linked directly with diminished sexual health and high-risk sexual decision-making among adolescent girls. And if that's not enough, frequent exposure to media images that sexualize girls and women has been proven to lead to stronger endorsement of sexual stereotypes that depict women as sexual objects and that value women primarily for their physical attractiveness. Yuck.

The APA hypothesizes that, although most of these studies have been conducted on women in late adolescence, findings are likely to generalize to younger adolescents and to girls, who may be even more strongly affected because their sense of self is still being formed. It also acknowledges the profound effect of pervasive sexualized images of girls and women on boys and men, who may hold sexist beliefs, have unrealistic ideals of female sexual attractiveness, and see women as playing a secondary role in relationships (and in society in general). Yikes.

There's no simple solution, but the good news is that we can mitigate the effects of hypersexualization by teaching our kids from a young age to be media literate. Using open conversation, positive role modelling, teachable moments, and the suggestions in this (and the next) chapter, we can teach kids to think critically about what they see and hear in media. Only then will they be empowered to be their true selves online and in real life.

■ INTERMEDIATE CHECKLIST (GRADES 4 AND 5)

Your Grade 4 and 5 child needs to know everything the previous age groups have learned, plus
- the responsibilities that come with the decision to be in a sexual relationship
- basic information about sexually transmitted infections (STIs)
- more about the different ways that families are formed, and that all families (i.e. single parent, blended, divorced, gay, adoptive) deserve respect
- that homophobic and transphobic language, jokes, and attitudes are unacceptable

They should also have acquired
- knowledge about physical and emotional changes at puberty
- skills that foster a healthy body image
- basic assertiveness skills
- how to make smart decisions and stay safe on the Internet
- basic digital and media literacy, including an awareness of hypersexualization in media and pop culture

7. Managing Media and the Internet

7: Managing Media and the Internet

■ INTERMEDIATES (GRADES 6 AND 7)

It goes without saying that the conversations parents have had with their Grade 4 and 5 children about the Internet are even more important to repeat and review when their kids are in Grades 6 and 7.

MediaSmarts, which has performed several studies on the use of technology by Canadian kids, identifies age 13 as the time when most of them begin to develop "sophisticated" Internet skills – exactly the same time that they begin to crave more independence from their parents. MediaSmarts found that over 75% of the kids surveyed had the skills to delete their Internet history, and 30% admitted to doing so. Not to mention that most kids know all about parental-control software and how to get around it. Even if this weren't the case, we obviously can't put parental controls on every computer our children will come into contact with over their teen years. What we *can* do, though, is beef up our conversations about the Internet with our older intermediates.

Here's the thing. Even before they become teens, our kids are straddling two worlds: their "real" world, and their online world. And, as they get older, they want us parents to be less and less involved in both. They go to great efforts to make this happen, and if we parents think we can keep tabs on *everything* our preteens and teens are doing online, we're kidding ourselves. Teens are exceptionally good at hiding their tracks and they tell me that having multiple Facebook or Instagram accounts to do this is the oldest trick in the book. We talked in the previous chapter about the importance of parents following and being friends with their preteens and teens on social media from day one. But if they have multiple accounts, we're only catching a glimpse of their activity. So how would parents know if this is the case?

Rosalind Wiseman, author of *Queen Bees and Wannabes* and an internationally recognized expert on children and parenting, wisely suggests that if you see messages on your child's Facebook wall like, "Hey, where have you been?" or "Are you still using this account?" chances are they've set up a new one.

But even if our preteen *doesn't* have more than one account, the question is, "How much privacy should I give them?" and "Should I insist on knowing their passwords?" The short answer is, "Yes." Of course, they can change their password at any time without your knowledge, but it doesn't hurt to randomly ask them to log in every now and then while you're watching. Some parents question whether they have the right to access their child's social media accounts without their knowledge for fear of invading their privacy.

But here's the bottom line: we need to teach our kids, from the time they can pick up an iPad, that there *is* no privacy online. The Internet is a public space. If they want to share something privately with someone, they need to have a face-to-face or phone conversation. And parents, no fair to listen in. Journals and diaries are also off limits for us. Let's give our kids the privacy they need, but it can't be online.

This doesn't mean we should troll our preteen's social media accounts every night before bed. I agree with Wiseman that there are two situations that warrant us checking: when we're out of town and our preteen or teen isn't with us (social media is the party hotline and we need to know what they're up to in our absence), and if we're concerned that something's going on. Some parents tell me they have their child write down their password and put it in a sealed envelope taped to the fridge. The parent will only access the password should the need arise. Sounds to me like a good way to build and maintain trust.

BE SMART ABOUT SMART PHONES

Although I mentioned earlier that I don't believe there's any good reason for a child to have a smart phone before they go to high school, I'm including this section in this chapter because most Grade 6 and 7 students have them.

I was speaking with a parent one night after one of my sessions. She was torn as to whether or not she should get her 10-year-old daughter a smart phone before school started in September and wanted my opinion. When I asked her why her daughter would need one, the parent reasoned that she would just feel better knowing she had one walking home from school. My question was, if the walk home from school is so dangerous, shouldn't someone pick her up?

Other parents tell me they buy phones for their Grade 6 and 7 kids "to keep tabs on them." The truth is, unless "location services" is always on (and it can easily be turned off) there's no way of knowing *where* your child is. Gone are the days when calling them on a landline prevented them from telling you they were somewhere they weren't. A better way to keep track of your preteen or teen's whereabouts might be to stay in close contact with other parents. Check in with them before and during sleepovers, for example. I know one parent who often texts her son midway through a Saturday night and asks him to text her a photo of where he is, preferably with a date and time stamp. If he doesn't respond within an agreed upon time period, that's her go ahead to go out and find him.

As Wiseman warns, though, we have to make sure that we don't overuse our stealth investigative skills on our preteens and teens. We need to use technology strategically so that our preteens and teens are "slightly paranoid" that we can track their whereabouts, but not so paranoid that they take their sneakiness to the next level, or don't call us when they're in trouble for fear of the consequences. In short, Wiseman suggests, "When you have a teenager, your goal is to keep one step ahead of them. This has been and always will be the goal. Likewise, teens will always be looking for the next way to get one over on you. Don't take it personally. And remember, a small degree of fear and paranoia can literally save your child's life."

When it comes to knowing your preteen's phone password and reading texts, I do recommend you monitor the phone bill so you'll notice any excessive texts being sent and received by their phone, especially late at night. Hopefully, they're respecting the no-phones-in-bed rule and it's not an issue. But sleeping with their phone is problematic for a few reasons. First, if they're texting all night, they aren't sleeping and will be a basket case at school the next day. Decreased

---

TEXT DICTIONARY

(From CNN's special report *Being 13: Inside the Secret Life of Teens*, hosted by Anderson Cooper)
1. OOTD – Outfit of the day.
2. KOTD – Kicks of the day – Typically refers to sneakers.
3. HMU – Hit me up – Usually asking for someone's Snapchat username, a phone number to text, or for a direct message.
4. Smash – I would have sex with you – A girl might post a provocative picture and a boy might write "smash."
5. Cook session – When one or several teens gang up on another kid on social media.
6. TBH – To be honest – A teen might post a picture of himself or herself and ask for a TBH, usually looking for positive responses.
7. TBR – To be rude – While TBH often leads to positive responses, TBR is usually followed by a negative response.
8. OOMF – One of my followers – A secretive way to talk about one of their followers without saying their name, such as "OOMF was so hot today."
9. BAE – Baby – affectionate term for someone's girlfriend, boyfriend, etc.
10. WCW – Woman Crush Wednesday – A girl will post a picture of another girl she thinks is pretty, while guys will post pictures of girls they think are hot.
11. MCM – Man Crush Monday – Similar to Woman Crush Wednesday, but featuring pictures of men.
12. BMS – Broke my scale – A way to say they like the way someone looks.
13. RDH – Rate date hate – As in "rate me, would you date me, do you hate me?" A typical response might be "rate 10 date yes hate no" or "10/y/n."
14. IDK – I don't know.

melatonin in the body as a result of looking at the screen doesn't help the situation either. Second, although friendly banter between friends late into the night is fun, what if the banter isn't friendly at all? Sleeping hours may be your child's only real escape from the bullying or harassment they've been dealing with all day.

Especially as they move toward high school, we should teach our preteens the value of unplugging and not being slaves to our smart phones. For example (although not always easy or successful), in my family we've tried to carve out smart-phone-free time over the years. We don't have phones at the table during meal times *ever* and, for the most part, our devices are all charging in a designated area of the kitchen by 10 p.m. I know, don't we sound perfect? Well, we're not. When we're on vacation at a restaurant, all four of us are guilty of pulling out our phones while waiting for our food. One minute you're just checking the weather for the next day and before you know it you're knee deep in Instagram. And because one of my stepdaughters is less glued to social media (and her phone in general), we don't always know where her phone is at 10 p.m. The point is, we can set expectations and goals for smart, smart phone use that we all benefit from.

It can also be tough for parents to put the device away if they're relying on it to entertain their child, or if it gives them a few minutes of serenity while visiting with a friend. If a child is at a dinner party with only adults, I don't blame them for wanting to bury their face in an online game. But (almost) nothing is more irritating than being introduced to a friend's child and they don't even look up from their iPad to acknowledge you. Not only is this incredibly rude, but the child is deprived of learning important social skills and basic manners. I worry that this will have an impact (and already has had) on how our kids learn to interact with others. Text and email are great, but nothing can replace face-to-face interaction. A child who's constantly on a device at social events won't have a clue how to handle an in-person job interview in high school, or have a conversation with their partner's parents someday. We're doing our kids a huge disservice if we aren't teaching them good manners around devices.

■ WE LIVE IN A **SELFIE SOCIETY**

You don't have to be a sociologist to know that our society has quickly developed an obsession with the *selfie*, a photo that someone has taken of themselves, typically with a smart phone and shared via social media. Please know that I'm not here to say that selfies are evil. They can be fun for people of all ages, and if shared, positive comments and likes give us a boost. It's human nature. And, especially for preteens and teens, seeking validation in this way is a totally normal, healthy way to develop self-identity.

But it's a slippery slope. Particularly for girls, self-esteem can quickly become reliant on "comments," "likes," and "follows" based purely on image and appearance (external factors), rather than on personality, talents, or smarts (internal factors). Rather than just offering friends a snapshot into someone's daily life, selfies can become a desperate plea: "Tell me I'm pretty," or "Look how funny and cool I am." If someone gets a positive response ("Gorge!"), that can make for a good day. Negative responses ("Get over yourself.") can ruin several days.

Or, if a selfie is posted and responses don't start pouring in right away, one might immediately ask, "Why isn't anyone liking my post?" or "Did I use the wrong filter?" or "Does this mean I'm ugly?" In minutes, self-doubt takes over, they delete the post, and then try again. As a stepmother of girls, I worry that if one selfie didn't get the response they were looking for, the next selfie might be a bit more attention getting…maybe a bit more edgy, provocative, sexy? And that's dangerous territory for a preteen girl.

So how can we help our kids (and some of our adult friends) find the balance needed to have a healthy relationship with selfies? Lots of preteens and teens already do. But parents might want to check in with their intermediate child and get them to ask themselves some of these questions.

■ "Is taking selfies getting in the way of me being where I am at that moment?" Focusing on taking photos can very easily result in missing a fun, meaningful, or interesting experience.

- "Am I doing this for fun, or do I *need* the comments and likes?" At iGirl (the empowerment workshop I and my team of educators offer to girls aged 9–12), we compare self-esteem to a fire inside us. If we rely on likes and comments as fuel, we can only keep the fire going for so long...eventually, we'll run out because we're depending on others to provide it. If we fuel our fire from within by recognizing our uniqueness, celebrating our talents and special qualities, and telling ourselves we matter, our fire will never go out.
- "Am I posting selfies in moderation, or is it overkill?" Sometimes less is more.
- "Is this selfie interesting, important, or inspirational to others?" Photos that document activities and experiences are way more interesting than a new clothing purchase, or what you're eating for lunch.

The bottom line is that, as parents, we want selfies to be a positive and empowering aspect of our kids' lives. The key message is this: have fun posting selfies, but don't let external gratification control you. And remember that the purpose of social media is to help us connect and feel good, not to stress us out and trash our self-esteem!

BYSTANDERS CAN BEAT CYBERBULLYING

As its name indicates, social media is meant for socializing. For the most part, young people's interactions online are positive. More and more, though, social media is being used as a platform for abuse, harassment, intimidation, and threats, also known as cyberbullying. In fact, MediaSmarts reports that roughly one-quarter of young people report having been targets of cyberbullying. And, not surprisingly, one-third of students who were bullied online reported symptoms of depression, a figure that rose to nearly one-half for those who experienced both online and offline bullying.

Cyberbullying is different from face-to-face bullying in few ways. First, it can be more intense and cruel because the Internet provides anonymity. Even if a bully isn't anonymous, people are a lot braver when they can type instead of having to say something mean to a person's face and see their hurt reaction. Plus, without hearing the tone of voice and seeing other non-verbal cues, comments intended as jokes may be misinterpreted. Second, the audience for cyberbullying is so much larger. Instead of just a few people hearing an insult on the playground, thousands of people can read it on social media in a matter of minutes.

Third, there's no escape for victims of cyberbullying. Gone are the days when a child could come home to a safe haven after recesses and lunches of bullying at school. Online harassment is relentless and comes in 24/7. Other than blocking a person's messages, the only escape is to turn your phone off. For a preteen or teen, this could lead them to feel even more excluded, missing out on positive interactions with their friends just when they need them most.

iMatter is our workshop for preteens aimed at inspiring respect online among youth. A big chunk of the program is spent offering participants tips on how they can make this happen. Here are a few that parents may find helpful when discussing cyberbullying with their intermediates. Just to clarify the lists below, "iMatter Nevers" refer to things that we should *never* do online. Likewise, "iMatter Musts" refer to things that we should *always* do online.

■ IMATTER NEVERS

I must never...

■ reply aggressively to a bully – that makes me a bully, too. Plus, online bullies are just like real life ones; they want me to answer and give them a reaction so that they feel powerful.

■ make assumptions about who did/said what online.

■ make assumptions about someone's character based on a rumour or actions.

- ask someone to send a sexual photo to me online or by text.
- post or send a sexual photo of myself online or by text.
- forward a sexual photo that someone has sent me online or by text.
- ask someone to do something online that I wouldn't feel comfortable doing myself.
- threaten someone online.
- participate in hate websites or groups (that includes not doing anything to shut them down).
- underestimate the power I have to help someone cope with online harassment.
- assume that someone else is going to help a victim of harassment.

■ IMATTER MUSTS

I must...

- treat others how I would like to be treated. (It sounds cliché, but it's true!)
- use abbreviations (such as JK or LOL for joking) to express myself more clearly online so my message is less likely to be misinterpreted.
- block a bully's messages.
- save any harassing messages and make a report to my Internet Service Provider (most have policies restricting harassment).
- remember that not doing anything when someone is being harassed sends the message that I think it's okay. Just my presence (online or in person) makes me part of the problem, if I don't take a stand.
- have empathy for a victim of harassment, even if I don't know them. I must put myself in their shoes.
- do what I can to make the situation better (talk to the bully, report). I must use social media in a positive way to spread the word that cyberbullying isn't okay.
- go to the source. If someone has said or done something to me, I must talk to them in person. Face-to-face conversations are always better than online conversations, especially in difficult times. Be assertive.

- advocate for ways to report cyberbullying anonymously at my school, if they aren't in place already.
- leave a chat room, game, or website if I'm being harassed.
- remember that saying something mean online is, in many ways, more cruel than saying it in person because it reaches so many people over and over again.
- remember the positive influence I can have on a younger sibling, or on someone who looks up to me. They're watching and listening to everything I do and say, looking to me for guidance.
- reach out to someone if I know they're being harassed…even just standing beside them is powerful.
- remember that uttering threats, impersonating someone, and sending sexual photos online without consent is against the law.
- print harassing messages and keep a log.
- use the support of my friends, parents, teachers, or other trusted adults.
- be socially responsible, even when the victim of cyberbullying may not be someone I know.

On that last point, bear with me while I tell you about an experience I had with this as an adult. I'm Facebook friends with an old family friend, a male who's 26 years old. (Let's call him Kevin.) I haven't been in touch with Kevin for years, but it's been fun reconnecting with him on online as adults. A couple of years ago, I came across one of his posts and found it extremely offensive. It was a photo of a girl passed out in front of a building that looked like a bar, and the way she was lying on the ground showed a glimpse of her underwear. Even more disturbing than this degrading photo were the 25 or so comments below it, for example, "Hey, Kevin, your girl needs new underwear!" with him responding, "I don't date scum."

I felt so many different things after reading the comments, but mostly I couldn't believe that someone I knew could degrade, humiliate, harass, and judge someone they didn't even know. For entertainment. After thinking about it for a day or so, I private messaged Kevin, telling him as respectfully as I could how his post made me feel, knowing that there was a good chance he would just de-friend me and that would be it. That was a risk I was willing to take, but to my surprise he responded a couple of days later. Through several messages back and forth, he took responsibility for posting the photo, and acknowledged that what he did was *not okay*. I don't want to take too much credit, but I do believe that Kevin will think twice before posting in the future. I feel like I made a difference, and I was proud to share the story with my stepdaughters.

■ SEXTING SAVVY

Just so we're all on the same page, the term *sexting* (Yes, it's now in the dictionary!) refers to the act of sending someone sexually explicit photographs or messages via cell phone. Parents, catch your breath while I share some good news. MediaSmarts reports that among those who own a cell phone, only 4% of Grade 8 students have sent a sext of themselves to someone. Based on that finding, the chances that your Grade 6 or 7 child is sexting are slim. This means that your conversation about sexting with your preteen is pretty much a preventative one, so let's keep it in perspective.

More good news is that there's no evidence that teens who engage in sexting are more likely to engage in sex in real life. For example, one recent study concludes that sexting and sexual behaviour in adolescents are linked – in that it's common for youth to send sexually explicit texts or emails while they are exploring their budding sexuality – but not that sexting *leads to* sexual experimentation.

So what's the big deal, then? Many of us agree that the consensual sharing of sexual photos can be a way for people to create intimacy in their relationships and express themselves sexually. Not to mention there's no risk of sexually transmitted infections and unintended pregnancy in this type of interaction! And given that so much of teens' relationships exist online, sexting isn't too far out of the realm of possibilities. So yes, I'm all for healthy sexual exploration by people at all ages. At the same time, though, we want to protect our kids from possible harm. And this is what makes talking about sexting with young people tricky business. The reality is that sexting may have serious social, legal, and emotional consequences, particularly for teenagers, even with consent.

Before we get into the parenting stuff, let's look at Canadian laws around sexting. Until very recently, the sending of sexual images of a person under the age of 18 was considered distribution of child pornography, even when it was consensual. And most sexting images exchanged by teens qualify as child pornography, if there's nudity in the image. This means that the same laws used to punish adults distributing child pornography for the purpose of exploiting children were also being used to punish youth sharing sexual photos consensually with their partners.

Today, there's an exception set out in the Supreme Court of Canada (*R. v. Sharpe*) that may exclude the exchange of sexual images between intimate partners, provided that the sexual relationship is legal (it complies with age-of-consent restrictions) and the images aren't shared with other people. So if a 15-year-old girl sends a photo of her breasts to her 16-year-old boyfriend and it's not shared with anyone else, chances are the two of them will be protected by this exception to child pornography offences.

As of March 2015, it became illegal to non-consensually distribute sexual images, even if the subject of the photos is an adult. Because this offence is considered less serious, it's likely that teens who distribute sexual images of peers without their consent will be charged with this offence instead of child pornography offences.

Still, we as parents are wise to encourage our teens to express themselves sexually in a way that's safer and less permanent, at least until they're adults.

In addition to legalities, we need to consider the possible social and emotional consequences of sexting among youth. It doesn't take an Internet expert to know that once a photo is out there in cyberspace, there's no getting it back. Within minutes, a sexual photo can be seen by thousands of people via social media, email, or text, possibly causing the sender shame and humiliation. And because the majority of high school relationships are short-lived, a sexual photo intended as a private gift for one's partner can very quickly become a photo of an ex- used to get revenge or for retaliation. And the reality is that teens don't always have the best judgment when emotions take over. (Nor do some adults, for that matter!)

In the long term, we also worry that future employers and university admissions officers might make assumptions about a person's character based on what they find online. We would hate for a young adult to miss out on an opportunity because of a photo they or someone else posted years earlier. It's difficult for a teen to think about such long-term effects, but we need to stress the permanence of anything posted online.

> *If you like someone and they ask you for a nude and you don't wanna send it but you don't want them to dislike you... what would you say?*

Something else to consider is the motivation behind sending a sext. It's one thing for a sexual photo to be shared with someone if it was the sender's idea, they feel totally comfortable with it, and they're confident it will be used for the enjoyment of only the person it was intended for. Among adults, researcher Andrea Slane calls this "good sexting." But what if a person has been threatened, pressured, or coerced into sending a sexual photo of themselves? Not okay, and this is what we're working to prevent.

We also can't ignore that it's usually girls who are the senders of sexts, with boys more likely to be the receivers. This places girls at increased risk. In a world where sexism and double standards between the sexes still rule, a sexual photo described by one person as sexy can very quickly be judged by others as slutty. And this ridicule, shaming, and harassment can happen even if the photo in question was shared without consent. On the other hand, a guy who shares a sexual photo sent to him is branded by his peers as a stud, stallion, a pimp, or a player: all compliments in his world. This reflects discriminatory gender stereotypes that are still alive and well today. Girls are taught to protect their sexual innocence and purity; boys are taught that their sexual conquests are something to brag about.

So how do we talk about these concerns in a meaningful but not preachy way with our preteens and teens? The most productive conversations we can have with our kids about sexting (or anything, really) are ones that offer insight and ask questions free of judgment. Here are some suggestions.

Be proactive. Don't wait until an incident has occurred to talk about sexting. Preload your child with information and discussions before high school so that their decisions online are well-informed. Ask general questions and position them as the expert: **"Do you think many people your age are sexting, or are we parents freaking out for no reason?"** If sexting is already an issue for your child, listen without judgment before jumping into problem-solving mode.

If your child has sexted and it's been shared, now is not the time for, "I thought you knew better!" Let them know you support them 100% and will help them find the courage to go to school the next day. Practice some assertive responses to any teasing they might experience. Save the, "What were you thinking?" talk for later. It's important to have, but wait until the dust settles.

Brainstorm healthy forms of sexual expression and exploration. What activities are age-appropriate, consistent with your values, and in your comfort zone? In Grades 6 and 7, maybe flirty texts and smooches behind the bleachers are fun and harmless.

Talk about the permanence of the Internet. Even if a photo is sent to one person privately, it can easily and quickly be shared through social media, email, text, or a screen shot. And once a photo is in cyberspace, it's there for good.

Talk about the motivation behind sexting. **"Why do teens do it?" "Is it a positive, fun experience for them?" "Is it liberating and empowering to share intimacy this way with another person?" "Are there clear agreements around privacy and sharing of the photo?" "Can a person feel pressured to do it?" "What would be considered exploitative or abusive?"**

Stress that it's never okay for someone to pressure, threaten, or coerce another person to send a sext, even if they're in a relationship with this person. Partners in a healthy relationship show respect for each other's personal values and boundaries. If one person isn't comfortable doing something, it doesn't matter if their partner understands or not. They need to accept it.

Talk about the double standard when it comes to the outcomes of sexting for girls versus boys. **"Why is it that a girl who sends a sext risks being branded as a slut?" "And why is it that a boy who forwards to his friends a sext he has received is a pimp and a player and a stud?" "Is this fair?" "How can we change it?" and "Does this double standard exist in other aspects of our society?" "Do boys send sexts very often?"**

Help your child understand the laws around sexting. Sexual photos shared only between two consenting individuals are legal at any age, but that doesn't mean it's a good idea. We need to shift the focus to reflect the real crime: not the sexting itself, but the sharing of the photo without consent.

Remind your child that they should *never* pass on a sexual photo sent to them, even with consent. And if they pass a photo on without consent, it's against the law.

▌ PORNOGRAPHY ISN'T REAL

Loosely defined, pornography is material (usually images or video) that depicts sexual activity and that is intended to cause sexual excitement. When I bring up the topic of pornography with parents of preteens, they look both terrified and relieved to be talking about it. No surprise, pornography might just be the most daunting but also most important of all sexual health topics we need to tackle with our Grade 6 and 7 kids today.

You may be thinking, "My kid's only 11! Do we have to talk about this *now?*" Like everything else when it comes to sexual health, knowledge is power and prevention is key. And to those who are thinking, "Not my kid!" don't assume your teenager is exempt. If you consider your child to be an average kid, there's a pretty good chance they've watched porn.

In one survey of more than 5,000 Canadian high school students across all provinces and territories, 60% of Grade 9 and 10 boys admitted to having visited porn sites within the current academic year. That same study found that only 22% of kids had ever discussed online porn with their parents. A University of Alberta study found even more alarming figures: 90% of 13- and 14-year-old boys had watched porn at least once, and the majority of those visits were not the result of accidental clicks. (Teenage girls watch porn too, but the rate of consumption is higher for boys.)

In a perfect world, we'd figure out a way to prevent our preteens from being exposed to pornography. But in reality what we *can* do is

> Why do boy's feel like watching porn?
>
> why do girls when they have sex scream?
>
> What happens if you watch porn at a young age?

teach our kids to be porn literate, and to think critically about what they see in porn. Damage control, if you will. Here are some talking points that I've found work well, both in the classroom and at home.

I always start out my conversations with young people by stressing that pornography isn't bad or necessarily harmful. In fact, for a lot of people it makes masturbation and sexual relationships with others more fun and exciting. It can be perfectly healthy and arousing for adults to watch. But because it's adult material, it's against the law in Canada for people under the age of 18 to access or watch it. Pornography involving animals, children, or violence is illegal for everyone, no matter how old you are.

It's not real. Watching pornography and believing that's what a typical, healthy, meaningful sexual relationship looks like would be like watching an action movie and believing that it reflects how things happen in day-to-day life. In real life, sex is not always loud and dramatic. Rather, it's often quiet, peaceful, awkward, and boring to watch. Right, parents?

The actors in pornography may look like they're super aroused, but they're working. It's a job. They may *act* like they're having the time of their lives, but often what they're thinking is "When's my lunch break?" On this point, we have to be careful not to talk in a way that imposes judgment on this choice of work.

Pornography rarely depicts a typical healthy person's body. That is, most women do not have giant, perky, symmetrical watermelons for breasts. And men don't typically have 10-inch long penises that can shoot sperm six feet. Knowing this, it would be a waste of time to compare our bodies to theirs. It's also interesting that porn today almost always features hairless people, even male actors. This is a direct reflection of our culture's view that being hairless is sexier. Likewise, there's a glaring absence of cellulite, moles, and other skin imperfections. But what else is new?

[handwritten margin note: why do people have 12 inch dicks and watermelon breasts in porn?]

Pornography only represents one small (and sometimes extreme, exploitative, and disturbing) aspect of the complex experience a sexual relationship is. As well, if a young person feels aroused by watching an activity they know is violating, disrespectful, or just plain wrong, it can lead to feelings of shame and guilt.

Because (in research terms) it's a relatively new phenomenon, we don't yet know the long-term effects of watching online porn on young people. But how can it *not* affect their future sexual experiences in some way? I've met young men, for example, who've become so used to masturbating to pornography that they can't orgasm or even maintain an erection without it. Indeed, some experts are suggesting that men over the age of 50 who give up watching pornography can regain their sexual functioning faster than 20 year olds who give up watching pornography. They point to the plasticity of the young person's brain as a factor.

There may also be some confusion about what sexual consent

looks like in real life. In much of pornography, "no" means "yes," and we don't want our teens to think that's how real life works. We want our kids to have good, healthy, fun sex when they are adults, right? So addressing these concerns is a must.

Whenever I have the chance, I ask my students why they think teens watch pornography online. Interestingly, they tell me that curiosity is the motivating factor. We can't ignore the reality that most students aren't getting comprehensive sexual health education at school or from their parents. So we can't blame them for going online to get their questions answered.

Curiosity about sexuality and bodies is important and awesome, but pornography isn't a great way to learn. Again, porn is entertainment for the purpose of sexual arousal. And because the vast majority of preteens and teens have never been in a sexual relationship, what they see in porn can be confusing. Parents can suggest more productive ways of learning about sex and sexuality, such as exploring an educational website or app, getting some good sexual health books, or, even better, bringing questions to a trusted adult.

Feel free to break conversation about porn (and any other tough topic) into manageable chunks. It may be intense, and your preteen or teen may only be willing to engage you for short periods of time, like a one-way trip to lacrosse practice. But keep at it, and don't expect a "Thank you."

RESOURCES

FOR PARENTS

WEBSITES
- www.mediasmarts.com
- www.commonsensemedia.org
- www.mediatedreality.com
- www.safeonlineoutreachsociety.com
- www.uknowkids.com
- www.makelovenotporn.com
- www.loriboland.com (Hypersexualization of Youth Workshops)

BOOKS
- *Girls and Sex: Navigating the Complicated New Landscape*, by Peggy Orenstein.
- *Masterminds and Wingmen: Helping Our Boys Cope with Schoolyard Power, Locker-Room Tests, Girlfriends, and the New Rules of Boy World*, by Rosalind Wiseman.
- *Odd Girl Out: Revised and Updated: The Hidden Culture of Aggression in Girls*, by Rachel Simmons.
- *Queen Bees and Wannabes: Helping Your Daughter Survive Cliques, Gossip, Boyfriends, and the New Realities of Girl World*, by Rosalind Wiseman.
- *Talking to Your Kids about Sex: Turning "The Talk" into a Conversation for Life*, by Dr. Laura Berman.

ARTICLES
- *Sexting and the Law in Canada*, by Dr. Andrea Slane, in *Canadian Journal of Human Sexuality* 22, no. 3 (2013): 117–122.
- *Sexting and the Law* https://www.kidshelpphone.ca/Teens/InfoBooth/Sexting/Sexting-and-the-Law.aspx

FOR INTERMEDIATE CHILDREN

WEBSITES

- www.needhelpnow.ca (A site designed to provide information to youth who have been impacted by sexting)
- www.bullybeware.com
- www.safekidsbc.ca
- www.kidshelpphone.ca
- www.cyberbullying.ca
- www.thatsnotcool.com

ARTICLE

- "The Good, the Bad, and the Unexpected Consequences of Selfie Obsession," *Teen Vogue*, August 6, 2013. http://www.teenvogue.com/story/selfie-obsession

8. Sexual Consent and Gender Stereotypes

8. Sexual Consent and Gender Stereotypes

■ INTERMEDIATES (GRADES 6 AND 7)

■ CONSENT IS SEXY

By Grades 6 and 7, our kids would ideally have a pretty good grasp of what healthy consent looks and sounds like in their interaction with others. At this age, they probably understand the concept in terms of giving permission (for example, a parent giving their child consent to go on a field trip). Hopefully, they've also learned the importance of getting a person's consent before taking and sharing photos on social media. But what about *sexual* consent? How do we kick it up a notch and explain *that* to our preteens?

When I'm in the classroom with intermediates, one of the most relevant examples I use to illustrate the importance of sexual consent involves the "games" that teachers tell me they see happening at recess and lunch. These games feature butt-slapping, nipple twisting, and (boys) hitting each other in the genitals. Boys think girls like the attention. Girls tell me they hate it and would never consent to being slapped on the butt by a boy. Boys also tell me the last thing they find fun is to get hit in the testicles, but fear they'll be harassed by their peers if they don't participate or, even worse, report it. We need to help the instigators of these games understand that they're not okay. If anyone involved hates the game or doesn't consent, it's not a game at all. It's assault. Plus, they hurt and can be harmful to the body.

Because many young people have their first romantic relationships at this age, talking about sexual consent in this context is also relevant to Grade 6 and 7 kids. Even if your preteen isn't in a relationship or interested in one anytime soon, this is a good time to start having general conversations. For example, you could ask questions about relationships while watching TV together. **"How do you think he knew that she was into him?" "Did he ask her if she wanted him to kiss her?" "What if she asked to kiss him and he said 'No'?"** (Note that these questions intentionally refer to heterosexual relationships as mainstream TV shows don't feature homosexuals being physically intimate.)

> What do you do if you don't give someone sexually consent and they don't listen?

News stories about sexting also offer plenty of teaching opportunities. **"How would it feel to have a sexual photo of you shared with others without your consent?" "What would you do if you received a sexual photo that wasn't intended for you?"**

Helping preteens understand and manage their hormones is part of teaching sexual consent too. Explain that during puberty all people experience changes in hormones that affect emotions and urges, including sexual ones. These changes are perfectly healthy and normal, but they're your responsibility and no one else's. No matter how strong your feelings are, it's never okay to express affection or sexual attraction to someone in a way that might make them feel uncomfortable, or even worse, violated.

When it comes to sexual activity of any kind, preteens need to know exactly what sexual consent is and isn't. By having the conversation now, the information is preventative, and respectful habits are formed long before your child enters a sexual relationship. If we're going to come even close to creating a society free of sexual abuse and exploitation, we need to start talking about sexual consent early. Only then can we build a culture that demands respect for one another. Of course, we need to be good role models ourselves when it comes to this. Demonstrate healthy, respectful communication in your own relationships and point it out in relationships around you.

My wise colleague Heather Corinna is the creator of an invaluable sexual health website for teens and young adults called Scarleteen. One of my favourite articles on the site is entitled "Driver's Ed for the Sexual Superhighway: Navigating Consent." It gives the most comprehensive, youth-friendly discussion of sexual consent I have ever come across, so rather than reinvent the wheel, here's some of what Scarleteen has to say. Sexual consent is

an active process of willingly and freely choosing to participate in sex of any kind with someone else, and a shared responsibility for everyone engaging in, or who wants to engage in, any kind of sexual interaction with someone. When there is a question or invitation about sex of any kind, when consent is mutually given or affirmed, the answer on everyone's part is an enthusiastic "yes."

So what exactly does that mean? Well, "willingly and freely choosing" means that both partners are making sexual decisions in a safe, respectful environment in which they have equal power. They don't feel pressured or manipulated, and are comfortable with the outcomes of their decision.

"An enthusiastic yes" reflects a strong desire that a person wants to act on. They aren't indifferent or on the fence. There are many ways to express a "yes," but the safest and clearest way to do it is with words. Consent is best when it's a verbal, enthusiastic "YES!" Now *that's* sexy.

Perhaps most important, sexual consent isn't just a one-time thing that lasts for the duration of a relationship. It's fluid; it can be retracted and has to be mutual. Even sexier!

So what does this all mean for us as parents of preteens and teens? Scarleteen does a great job of highlighting the must-have information for people of all ages about this complex concept. Here's the *Coles Notes* version (*CliffsNotes*, if you're reading this in the U.S.)!

THE ESSENTIAL RULES OF THE CONSENSUAL ROAD

Sexual consent is about everyone involved in a sexual or possibly sexual interaction. For sex to be totally consensual, everyone needs to seek consent, everyone needs to give it, and everyone needs to accept and respect each other's answers.

Consent can *always* be withdrawn. So just because someone consented to sex on Tuesday doesn't mean they are also consenting to sex on Thursday and Saturday.

> *[handwritten]: What could happen if you have sex before 16.*

Consent is *never* automatic, unnecessary, or owed. Even being someone's spouse, boyfriend or girlfriend doesn't give the other person consent by default. Just because someone loves you, or says that they love you, doesn't mean you have their sexual consent, or that they have yours. Also, consenting to one kind of sex doesn't mean a person consents to any other kind of sex. For example, someone who engages in oral sex is not necessarily asking for, or consenting to, vaginal sex; someone who is cool with kissing is not necessarily cool with any other kind of touching.

If someone is drunk, high, passed out, asleep, or unable to truly understand what they are saying yes to, full, informed and free sexual consent *cannot* be given.

Non-consent means STOP. If someone is not consenting to something or says no with their words and/or actions, the other person *MUST* stop trying to do that thing *and MUST* not try to convince that person to do that thing in any way. If the person asking for sex doesn't stop, or if they exert emotional or physical pressure and the other person gives in, they are sexually assaulting that person. End of story.

And, for the record, a lack of "No" does not mean "Yes."

Sexual consent is actually pretty straightforward once you break it down into what it is and what it isn't. In terms of conveying this information to a preteen or teen, there's lots of help for parents online. For example, Laci Green, a peer sex educator with a frank YouTube video series about sexuality (she is truly a gift to young people everywhere), echoes these points in her "Wanna Have Sex? (Consent 101)" episode. It's only six minutes long, and definitely worth watching. If you have teens, make them watch it with you; I promise they'll find it so entertaining they won't even realize it's educational!

Another one of my favourite consent teaching tools, which is also on YouTube, is "Consent: It's Simple as Tea." It's short and hilariously logical.

> **Consent and the Law in Canada (Excerpted and adapted from information posted by the Government of Canada's Department of Justice)**
>
> **All sexual activity without consent, regardless of age, is a criminal offence. The age of consent refers to the age at which a young person can legally consent to sexual activity. The age of consent laws apply to all forms of sexual activity, ranging from sexual touching (e.g., kissing) to sexual intercourse. Raised from 14 years on May 1, 2008, the age of consent for sexual activity in Canada is 16 years.**
>
> **The *Criminal Code* provides "close in age" or "peer group" exceptions. For example, a 14- or 15-year-old can consent to sexual activity with a partner as long as the partner is *less than five years older* and there is no relationship of trust, authority, or dependency or any other exploitation of the young person. This means that if the partner is five years or older than the 14- or 15-year-old, any sexual activity will be considered a criminal offence unless it occurs after they are married to each other. There is also a "close-in-age" exception for 12- and 13-year-olds: a 12- or 13-year-old can consent to sexual activity with another young person who is *less than two years older* and with whom there is no relationship of trust, authority, or dependency, or other exploitation of the young person.**

Just before we claim ourselves and our intermediates to be sexual consent experts and move on, let's not forget two critical aspects of any meaningful discussion about sexual consent: the effects of gender stereotypes and how we define masculinity within a context of rape culture in our society. I know, it's a mouthful, but until we break down these gender stereotypes, sexual non-consent (assault) will continue to exist. Let me explain.

■ GENDER STEREOTYPES AND SEXUAL CONSENT

One of my proudest moments in 16 years of teaching happened during our first iGuy Empowerment Workshop pilot program in January 2014. At the end of the two-hour session, our facilitator, Andrew Shopland, asked participants to share with the group something about themselves that their peers may not know. When it came to his turn, one of the quieter boys in the class said, "Everyone thinks I'm all about sports, but I really enjoy sewing too."

Trying not to be obvious, Andrew and I looked at each other with tears in our eyes (seriously). It was in that moment that we knew we were on to something with iGuy. Given that a main goal of iGuy is to encourage boys to challenge gender stereotypes, we also reflected after the session that if every preteen boy were this courageous, there would be little need for the program!

At iGuy, we explain gender stereotypes in terms of two boxes: the Pink Box and the Blue Box. As you've probably already guessed, the Pink Box teaches girls how they have to act and how they have to "be" in order to meet society's definition of what it means to be a "real" girl.

According to the Pink Box, girls should
- like to wear dresses and play with Barbies
- be over-emotional (hence the term "drama queen")
- ask for help and support when needed (which is a lot)
- be nice, not ruffle anyone's feathers (be people pleasers)
- apologize even if they haven't done anything wrong
- allow boys and men to take the driver's seat in relationships

> • What is the best way to say "No"?

- spend a good chunk of their time focusing on their appearance, mostly so that they can get attention from boys
- not look too sexy, or they risk being branded as sluts.

The Blue Box teaches boys how they should act and "be" in order to meet society's definition of what it means to be a "real" guy. In addition to teaching them that they should love sports, list blue as a favourite color, and play with action figures, the Blue Box teaches boys they should

- be tough, strong and stoic even when they don't feel it
- be into girls (because if not, they're gay*)
- be stylish but not too stylish or try too hard to be stylish (because that means they're gay*)
- keep their emotions bottled up (because sharing them is girlie and gay*, a sign of weakness)
- be self-reliant (asking for support shows weakness).

The Blue Box also teaches that
- vulnerability is weakness
- it's okay to get what they want (and solve conflict) using violence, aggression, and power over others
- it's okay to have power over girls in relationships
- sexual conquests give them status among peers (sexual prowess is expected and rewarded)
- they are superior to girls.

* It's important to note that, according to the Blue Box, being "gay" not only refers to sexual attraction, but also means that a guy is like a girl in some way (weak, emotional, stylish).

■ AND THE LIST GOES ON.

And, according to the Blue Box, being a girl is pretty much the worst thing you could be. Looking at it this way, homophobia is really an extension of misogyny. Now there's an *Aha!* moment. But not in a good way.

I know it doesn't sound like it from the description above, but the Blue Box is not all bad, and some boys feel very comfortable living in it. It's incredibly limiting for most boys, though, in that it prevents them from being who they really are. As well, it reinforces a belief in hierarchy, which leads to bullying and other systems of oppression, such as rape culture.

Rape culture is caused by gender stereotypes that sanction the notion that boys are sexual predators and girls their sexual prey. Emilie Buchwald, author of *Transforming a Rape Culture*, describes that when society normalizes sexualized violence, it creates rape culture, which she defines as

a complex set of beliefs that encourage male sexual aggression and support violence against women. It is a society where violence is seen as sexy and sexuality as violent. In a rape culture, women perceive a continuum of threatened violence that ranges from sexual remarks to sexual touching to rape itself. A rape culture condones physical and emotional terrorism against women as the norm... In a rape culture both men and women assume that sexual violence is a fact of life, inevitable... However... much of what we accept as inevitable is in fact the expression of values and attitudes that can change. (from www.wavaw.ca)

The website Upsetting Rape Culture (www.upsettingrapeculture.tumblr.com) explains how rape culture is the result of images, language, laws, and other everyday phenomena that we see and hear every day and that validate and perpetuate rape.

Rape culture includes jokes, TV, music, advertising, legal jargon, laws, words and imagery, that make violence against women and sexual coercion seem so normal that people believe that rape is inevitable. Rather than viewing the culture of rape as a problem to change, people in a rape culture think about the persistence of rape as "just the way things are."

In order to change these values and attitudes, we need to reject the gender stereotypes that perpetuate male power over women. This starts with teaching our kids about not only about "power *over*," but also about "power *with*" and "power *within*", which is what we do in our iGuy workshops.

◼ THREE TYPES OF POWER

***Power over* is power taken from someone else, or from some other group.** Power over *imposes* authority over someone else. The rules of the Blue Box reflect society's *power over* boys. Bullying and sexual assault are classic examples of the consequences of believing in *power over*.

Power with reflects strength in numbers, an alliance to reach a common goal, earned through a sense of trust and community. Welcoming and standing up for others who don't fit into the Blue Box is *power with*.

Power within (**agency**) is an inherent feeling of self-worth, the ability to act with integrity, without relying on external approval or reinforcement. The iGuy participant who wasn't afraid to be vulnerable (revealing in front of his peers that he likes to sew, a hobby that certainly doesn't fit into the Blue Box) showed immense power *within*, because it was such a courageous act to openly admit a deviation from the Blue Box.

The goal of *power with* and *power within* is equality. With equality, rape culture could not exist.

So how can parents play a role in turning rape culture into consent culture? As always in parenting, there are no easy solutions. But here are some suggestions to get you on the right track.

Talk to your son about the Blue Box (vs. the Pink Box) and the extent to which gender stereotypes dictate how we talk and behave. Discuss how limiting it is to live inside the Blue Box and how it affects others. Which aspects of themselves fit into the Blue Box and which don't? What if we just thought about ourselves as humans? How would the world be different?

Ask what qualities make a good human. Are these qualities different for boys and girls?

Talk about what masculinity means in our society. What does it mean to be a man? How can we redefine masculinity so that men and women are equal? How can we make it more inclusive of all types of boys and men?

Talk about femininity in our society. Why is it something that boys are socialized to avoid at all costs? What does it mean to be a woman? Could it be that feminine traits serve boys well, too?

Talk about the importance of expressing emotions, speaking our truth, and asking for help when we need it. Discuss the fact that this vulnerability isn't weakness; it's courage. Stress that it's perfectly normal to feel a range of emotions, but reacting aggressively isn't healthy for anyone.

Next time you're watching TV together, comment on whether male characters are being true to who they really are. Or are they slaves to the Blue Box? How is that working for them? How is that working for their relationships?

Be a good role model. As a parent, do you express your emotions regularly in a healthy way, or do you bottle them up and explode when the pressure gets to be too much? Dads, do you have any hobbies or interests that aren't stereotypically masculine? Do you make comments that unintentionally reinforce the rules of the Blue Box (for example, "Toughen up! Be a man! Don't be a wimp! Don't cry! Real men do/don't do that!")? Do you make comments or jokes that are disrespectful or degrading to women? Be honest.

Explain the three different types of power. Which type of power does the Blue Box encourage boys to have? Is this useful or healthy for boys? Is this useful or healthy for our society? On the other hand, what type of power are girls taught to value? How does this difference affect relationships between males and females?

Give examples of what *power within* looks like:
- doing an activity you enjoy regardless of what others think
- embracing your own style of clothing even if it's not trendy
- asking for help when you need it
- calling out someone on using homophobic language
- courageously expressing your vulnerability and emotions
- standing up for yourself or for someone who is being bullied, harassed, or assaulted

- resisting peer pressure to say or do something you know is wrong
- acting with integrity (your actions and words match your values and morals)
- acting in a way that is respectful to women
- never acting without consent in a sexual relationship.

Talk about relationships. All humans deserve healthy relationships based on honesty, equality, respect, and integrity. Don't settle for less.

Talk about consent. How would someone know when it's okay to kiss or touch someone in a sexual way? What if consent isn't given? How could drugs or alcohol affect a person's judgment? If they witnessed what could be an assault (for example, at a party) what should they do?

Stress that it is *never* the responsibility of the victim to prevent an assault. The message should be "Don't rape," not "Don't get raped." We all need to take responsibility for our actions, and it's not okay to blame someone else for something we've done.

■ RESOURCES

FOR PARENTS

WEBSITES

- www.upsettingrapeculture.com
- www.goodmenproject.com
- www.wavaw.ca (Women Against Violence Against Women)
- www.therepresentationproject.org (an organization that inspires individuals and communities to challenge and overcome limiting stereotypes)
- www.higherunlearning.com (an online space to explore what it means to be a man today)

BOOKS

- *Transforming a Rape Culture*, by Emilie Buchwald, Pamela Fletcher, and Martha Ross.
- *Daring Greatly* and other books and writings by Brené Brown.

FOR PRETEENS AND TEENS

BOOKS

- *S.E.X., second edition: The All-You-Need-To-Know Sexuality Guide to Get You Through Your Teens and Twenties*, by Heather Corinna.

WEBSITES, CAMPAIGNS, AND YOUTUBE CLIPS

- www.amysmartgirls.com – an organization founded by artist Amy Poehler dedicated to helping young people cultivate their authentic selves
- www.higherunlearning.com – an online space to explore what it means to be a man today
- http://everydayfeminism.com/2015/06/how-society-treats-consent

It's Simple as Tea https://www.youtube.com/watch?v=fGoWLWS4-kU
- https://www.youtube.com/user/lacigreen
- www.justice.gc.ca

ALWAYS #LIKEAGIRL CAMPAIGN
- www.always.com/en-us/about-us/our-epic-battle-like-a-girl

DOCUMENTARIES
- *Miss Representation*, by The Representation Project.
- *The Mask We Live In*, by The Representation Project.

9. Relationships, Sex, and Health

9. Relationships, Sex, and Health

■ INTERMEDIATES (GRADES 6 AND 7)

■ FIRST RELATIONSHIPS

It's not unusual for steady relationships to form at the end of elementary school. If you think about it, things haven't changed much since we were growing up. I vividly remember waiting endlessly for a boy in my Grade 7 class to ask me to "go around" (his friends assured me he was going to) only to find that he had asked someone else while I was at a volleyball tournament. I also remember the two of us being paired off for the couples skate at Stardust roller rink on Saturdays. And how could I forget Sarah and Ben walking around the playground holding hands when the supervision aides weren't there? They were so cool.

I also remember the drama surrounding our new-found romantic interests, and that hasn't changed much either. Crushes can be all consuming, and can destroy friendships.

The nature of young relationships is quite different today, though. First, preteens can't help but be influenced by the relationships they see in the media. Yes, we saw relationships on TV as well, but we watched Cliff and Clair Huxtable. Now our kids follow the Kardashians involved in an array of dysfunctional relationships. They also watch inane vampire shows that teach them true love comes with drama, tragedy, and angst. Not to mention these shows feature teenagers having more sex than adults ever do.

Second, many young relationships today begin and are sustained on smart phones, mostly through text or social media messaging. When I was growing up, it was all about talking on the phone. And any brave soul who dared to call me had to risk my dad answering. With the phone strategically bolted to the wall in the kitchen, there was little privacy and my parents usually had a good idea of who I was talking to, and for how long. In my house now, our landline barely ever rings. In fact, the girls' cell phones barely ever ring!

It's increasingly difficult for parents to be involved and to know what's going on in their kids' relationships. Not only that, but young relationships can progress at lightning speed without the nervousness of face-to-face interactions. Because of this reality, it's never been more important for parents to show an interest in and be involved in their kids' relationships as much as possible.

Backing up a couple of steps, parents would ideally have already started an ongoing conversation about what a healthy relationship looks like and feels like. This isn't giving our preteens permission to jump into the first opportunity that presents itself, but it's never too early for children to start thinking about what they would look for in a relationship, and how they would expect to be treated. At iGirl, we do a small group activity to explore just that. And they get it. Even nine-year-olds tell us that a healthy relationship involves things like respect, kindness, trust, good communication, support, compassion, common interests, thoughtfulness, cooperation, and fun. They also tell us that they would never want to be in a relationship involving abuse of any kind, extreme jealously, put downs, lying, selfishness, back-stabbing, fighting every day, or cheating. Can't argue with that!

The girls think it's hilarious when we suggest that a healthy relationship is HERI (pronounced "hairy"), which means that it is based on **H**onesty, **E**quality, **R**espect, and **I**ntegrity. Thanks to our always creative facilitator Brandy Wiebe for that brilliance! Breaking it down, we explain that honesty in a relationship means that partners always tell the truth, no matter how difficult it is. Equality means that both partners have equal say in the decisions they make. One person isn't the boss. Treating a partner with respect involves (among other things) listening to their concerns, honouring their boundaries, and showing consideration for their feelings. To act with integrity, in the context of a relationship, means that our actions are consistent with our beliefs. For example, a person who criticizes others for having affairs but then cheats on their partner is not acting with integrity. It's also worth pointing out that healthy *friendships* are HERI too.

Hands down, the best way we can teach our children what a healthy relationship looks like is to model one ourselves. Whether parents are married/partnered, divorced, dating, or single, our kids are learning from our relationships. Through our actions, we're showing them how to communicate, how to show affection, how to make decisions, and how to solve conflict. We always have to be mindful of this. Be honest with yourself: Do you bottle up emotions until you explode? Do you take responsibility for mistakes and apologize to your partner when warranted? Do you have difficulty expressing how you feel to your partner? How vulnerable are you in your relationship? Which of your qualities would you want/not want your child to have in their relationships?

> What should I do if I'm in a love triangel?

In her book *Talking to Your Kids about Sex*, therapist and sex educator Dr. Laura Berman echoes my suggestion that parents would ideally have already set some guidelines with their preteen before dating starts, based on their comfort level and family values. I remember my dad telling me once, as a child, "You can start dating when you're married!" At the time, that sounded pretty reasonable to me. Seriously, though, we don't want our preteens to think that dating rules are created as a knee-jerk reaction, or without much thought. Communicate them well ahead of time so there are no surprises. Berman suggests we ask ourselves, "At what age would I feel comfortable with my child starting to date?" Would these be group dates, or unsupervised one-on-one dates? And when is an appropriate age to have a steady relationship? You'll need to be flexible as your child gets older. For example, maybe group-dates-only is the rule for Grade 6 and 7, but in Grade 8 they can graduate to going unsupervised to a movie with someone they're dating.

Be sure to grab any chance you can to get to know their partner (but don't call them that unless they say you can!). Be interested, but not too interested. Invite them for dinner and on family outings. And if it looks like the relationship is going to last a while, get to know their parent(s). As difficult as it can be to get your head around your child being in a relationship, think of it as baby steps. Embracing and being involved as much as you can in these "beginner" relationships will make life a lot easier down the road, when your teen becomes interested in more serious dating.

And, very important, don't assume that your preteen or teen will be in a relationship with someone of the opposite sex.

[Handwritten note: How many ways of sex are there?]

■ SEX REDEFINED

Up to this point, explaining to children that the term "sexual intercourse" (or "sex") means that "the penis is inserted into the vagina" works pretty well. But if we're being honest, this definition refers specifically to *vaginal intercourse* (or *vaginal sex*), and we need to make the distinction for our preteens. Before going to high school, they need to understand that there are, in fact, many different types of sexual activity. Most of our kids *do* know this, but their information is usually coming from less-than-reliable sources. When I ask a typical group of Grade 6 and 7 students about the types of sex they have heard of (other than vaginal sex), they list the following, in this order. I start the discussion of sex by giving them scientific definitions for each term.

Blow jobs (oral sex):
Oral sex involves any kind of contact between the mouth and the genitals. The slang term "blow job" refers to oral sex performed on a person with a penis, and the scientific word for this is fellatio. The scientific word for oral sex performed on a person with a vulva and vagina is cunnilingus. Some people call it "going down."

Bum (anal) sex:
Anal sex involves the penis being placed in the anus.

Internet sex/cybersex:
Internet sex/cybersex involves people having a sexual interaction using technology, such as webcams, social media, text, or email.

Fingering (a type of digital or manual sex):
Digital sex involves hands or finger(s) stimulating the genitals or being placed inside genital openings.

Phone sex:
Phone sex involves people having a sexual interaction either by speaking on the phone or by text (also known as sexting).

Just so they know, I tell kids that *outercourse* is a general term used to refer to sexual activity that doesn't involve penetration; in other words, it doesn't involve body parts entering body parts: hugging, kissing, touching of genitals, intimate dancing, and massage are examples. Does anyone remember the term "heavy petting"? I can't say it or even type it with a straight face, but today it would be called outercourse.

I think it's also helpful to point out to Grade 6 and 7 kids that masturbation, also known as self-stimulation, is a type of sex. *Mutual masturbation* involves partners masturbating in front of each other or stimulating each other's genitals. It doesn't get much safer than that!

When talking about different types of sexual activity with Grade 6 and 7 students, it's not uncommon for them to ask, "How do gay people 'do it'?" I respond to this question by stressing that it's not like gay people "do it this way" and straight people "do it that way." Besides, what about all the people who don't identify with either of these two groups? Are they not allowed to have sex? Or do they have their own totally different way of having sex? The honest, scientific answer is that in a healthy relationship, consenting partners would decide *together* how they want to have sex, if at all, regardless of their sexual attraction. For obvious reasons, a cis-male gay couple wouldn't have vaginal sex. But a cis-male in a relationship with a trans male may. Both a gay and a straight couple may enjoy oral sex. One straight couple may choose to have anal sex, but another may not. And even some adults are surprised to hear that not all gay men enjoy anal sex.

Grade 6 and 7 students also ask me a lot of questions about slang terms when it comes to sex. Usually, the questions are written on pieces of paper and submitted anonymously. I don't feel the need to define every possible slang term they bring up in class, but it's worthwhile to explain those I hear on a regular basis. For example, many students at this age have heard slang terms for sexual positions, such as "69." I define this as any sexual position that allows partners to perform oral sex on each other at the same time. As you can imagine, the response I usually get is "Ewww! That is so disgusting!" to which I reply, **"That's how you're supposed to react! Most people your age aren't into oral sex. You may change your mind later, but don't worry about that now."**

> *Why would someone want to touch their mouth to another person's genital,*

One reason kids need to know the meaning of sexual slang terms is so that using these terms doesn't get them into trouble. A couple of years ago, I was at a school where a Grade 5 boy was meeting with the school's police liaison officer after reports that he'd been walking around the playground at recess telling girls that he wanted to "69" them. He told the officer that, at the time, he had no idea what the term meant; he had heard his older brother using the term in a conversation with a friend and wanted to see what kind of reaction he'd get from girls in his class. You can imagine his embarrassment and fear when he learned that what he was doing was actually considered sexual harassment, a serious crime with major consequences if charges had been laid.

It's also useful to define sexual slang for preteens because it takes away the word's power. For example, Grade 6 and 7 kids often ask me, "What's a douchebag?" This slang term has been recycled from when we were in high school to mean a jerk or a loser, among other things.

But when I explain to a group of Grade 7 boys in intricate detail the literal meaning of a douchebag (a vessel for vaginal cleansing fluid), all of a sudden it's not so cool to call their buddy that on the playground!

By the way, if you're child asks you the meaning of a slang word you've never heard of, (which is quite possible given that it's almost impossible to keep up with them all), tell them you'll report back in a few minutes. Then rush to your nearest device and search www.urbandictionary.com. I promise you'll find the answer to the question there.

■ VIRGINITY

While we're on the topic of slang, I think this is a good time to talk about the confusing concept of virginity. Students are asking me less and less often what virginity means, because we seldom use the term these days. But because it still comes up every now and then in the classroom, let's discuss it.

I think the concept of virginity is outdated and useless for several reasons. First, it's based on misinformation about anatomy. When I first started teaching in the late '90s, a virgin was simply defined as a person who had never had vaginal sex. It was also assumed that first-time vaginal sex would tear a woman's hymen and cause bleeding, and that if a woman didn't bleed the first time she had vaginal sex with her partner, then clearly she wasn't a virgin.

We know now that this isn't true. Some girls are born without a hymen, and some hymens get torn and are stretched painlessly and without bleeding long before sexual contact. Stories about women having their "cherry popped" the first time they have vaginal sex are garbage. That ugliness is much more about ignorance of anatomy than about virginity.

It's also worth letting our children know that no one, not even a doctor, can say with absolute certainty whether someone has or has not had vaginal sex. Of course, the presence of sperm or semen, STI organisms, or bruising and tearing in or around the vagina may be an indication of vaginal sex. But maybe not. Pregnancy can happen without penetration and so it isn't an indicator either.

I also have a problem with the concept of virginity because it's too simplistic. That is, it doesn't take into account the different kinds of sex a person may have, and makes the assumption that vaginal sex is the be-all and end-all. What if a person has never had or doesn't plan to have vaginal sex, but has had anal and oral sex? Are they a virgin their whole lives?

I also find the saying and the idea of "losing one's virginity" very sex negative. In a healthy, consenting sexual relationship, there's nothing to lose and lots to gain – like pleasure, intimacy, fun, stress relief, and physical and emotional connection with another human.

Lastly, I just don't get the point of the concept. Really, who cares if a person is a virgin? And if a person wants you to know about the kinds of sex they've had and haven't had, they'll tell you! End of story.

> *Handwritten note: If you're a girl can you lose your virginity to a girl.*

■ HOW MUCH SEX ARE TEENS HAVING, ANYWAY? (HINT: NOT MUCH)

No discussion of sex with preteens would be complete without helping them understand how many teens are, or aren't, sexually active in high school. When I ask kids to guess, Grade 6 and 7 students tell me they figure 80% to 90% of teens have had vaginal sex by the time they graduate. This isn't surprising given the ridiculous TV shows they watch, which feature heterosexual teenagers acting like they're in their 30s, the sexualized lyrics in music that lead them to believe that everyone's doing it, and the popularity of "reality" shows that give the impression that teen pregnancy is rampant. It gives me huge satisfaction to tell them they're wrong! Here's what we know from 2013 research surveying thousands of adolescents in British Columbia thanks to McCreary Centre Society's 2013 British Columbia Adolescent Health Survey (2013 BC AHS). I think you'll be pleasantly surprised.

Oral sex: In 2013, a total of 23% of students reported ever having oral sex, which was a decrease from 26% in 2008 for both males and females. Although equal percentages of males and females indicated having oral sex, males were more likely to have received oral sex (21% versus 18% of females), whereas females were more likely to have given it (21% versus 13% of males). Rates of both giving and receiving oral sex increased with age.

Vaginal sex: Preteens are especially surprised to learn that 81% of students in 2013 had never had vaginal sex. Only 19% of students indicated that they had ever had sex, other than oral sex or masturbation, with similar rates for males and females. This percentage reflected a decrease from a decade earlier for both genders (24% in 2003). Consistent with previous BC AHS findings and with the pattern for oral sex, older students were more likely than younger ones to have had vaginal sex. For example, 2% of Grade 7 students reported having had intercourse, compared to 44% of Grade 12 students.

You read that right. *Less than half* of high school graduates in British Columbia report having had vaginal sex. Now, I know that these statistics only show us part of the picture when it comes to the types of sex teens are having, and with whom. But at least when it comes to encouraging teens to delay vaginal sex, we must be doing something right!

When I ask Grade 6 and 7 students why teens are waiting longer these days to have sex for the first time, you can imagine the creative responses they come up with. I think my favourite came from a Grade 6 student who suggested it was because "the economy is weak." Most often, though, students tell me it's because, "They're scared of getting pregnant or getting an STI." While I'm always relieved to hear that those possible outcomes of sex are on their radar, even in elementary school, the last thing we want to do is *scare* young people out of having sex. There's a difference between being fearful and using information to make smart decisions. It's a good thing that young people today are more informed than *we* were growing up (not exactly earth shattering news given the poor puberty filmstrips that represented the extent of our sex education), but we can help our preteens and teens make smart decisions about sex with this information, without using fear as a motivating factor.

▰ HOW DO YOU KNOW YOU'RE READY FOR (ANY KIND OF) SEX?

With so much focus on pregnancy and STIs, it's easy to overlook the important emotional factors that play a role in sex-related decisions. But as young as Grade 4 and 5, students ask me, "When's a good age to have sex?" or "How do you know you're ready?" or "Do I ever have to do it?" There's no simple answer to any of these questions, but emotional readiness for any kind of sex deserves more attention than we tend to give it. When it comes to Grade 6 and 7 students knowing "when they're ready," the simple answer is, "Not any time soon!"

Now, I'm not suggesting that all sexual experiences involve a deep emotional connection that occurs in the context of a long-term, committed relationship. For many, a sexual experience is purely a physical connection with a partner and doesn't require soul-searching or a relationship evaluation. As long as the sex is consensual and the emotional and physical health of both partners is considered, then maybe it works. But still, the majority of sexual interactions between teens happen in the context of a relationship, and it's never too early to get preteens thinking about what they would expect and want in a relationship. I encourage kids to ask themselves these kinds of questions about a future sexual relationship.

- How compatible are we? Do we share similar values and goals?
- How long do I think this relationship is going to last?
- Would I be okay if we broke up after having sex?
- Can I be myself around my partner?
- Do I feel comfortable and safe with my partner?
- Am I hiding anything from my partner?
- Do I feel pressured by my partner? or my friends? or by society?
- What do my religious or family beliefs say about sex at my age?
- How would my parents feel if they knew? (How do they feel if they *do* know?)
- Do I feel proud of this relationship?
- How would I feel if people found out we were having sex?
- Is our relationship healthy?

In a healthy relationship, partners feel comfortable and safe expressing their boundaries clearly and honestly. They make sex-related decisions together and respect each other's choices. Each person acts with integrity, so clear boundaries are maintained without trying to convince their partner otherwise. And, of course, in a healthy relationship, all sexual activity is consensual.

Sounds very "Pleasantville," doesn't it? In a perfect world, our kids would carefully consider all of the above questions in discussion with us, before even contemplating sex of any kind. And they would only have sex within the context of an extremely HERI (Honest, Equal, Respectful and has Integrity) relationship. Too often, though, first sexual experiences are unplanned, minimally contemplated, alcohol or drug-fuelled events that didn't go anything like how a person imagined. But if we can preload our Grade 6 and 7 kids with some good information and important questions to think about, the odds are good that we can help them have a really positive first sexual experience.

TALKING ABOUT PREGNANCY AND CONTRACEPTION

Beyond emotional factors, we need to talk with our preteens about the physical responsibilities that come with each type of sexual activity, such as unplanned pregnancy and STIs. Of course, pregnancy as a possible outcome doesn't apply to all types of sex, nor does it apply to all sexual relationships. But let's remember that many preteens and teens are exploring their sexual attraction at this age and this may include experimentation with someone of the opposite sex, even if they identify as gay, or vice versa.

To be as sex-positive as possible, we need stress to our kids from day one that, **"In most circumstances, like between two consenting adults in a healthy relationship, sex is an intimate, pleasurable, stress-relieving, fun, awesome, special experience. And sex is probably going to be an amazing part of your life someday."** Now I know some of you are thinking, "Whoa, Saleema, let's be careful not to make sex sound *too* good to our kids!" The truth is, there's no such thing as enticing kids to have sex. First, most preteens and teens aren't interested in having sex anytime soon. Second, within this positivity around sex, we give them sound reasons to wait. Just before we talk about those reasons, here is some more good news from the 2013 survey I mentioned above.

PREGNANCY

Overall, 5% of youth who had had sexual intercourse reported having ever been pregnant or having caused a pregnancy in 2013, which was a decrease from 2008 (7%) and 2003 (6%).

CONDOM USE

In 2013, 69% of students who had had sexual intercourse reported that they or their partner had used a condom or other latex barrier the last time they had sex (72% of males versus 66% of females). When it comes to oral sex, 17% of students reported that they or their partner had used a condom or other barrier the last time they had engaged in it, with similar rates for males and females. However, this rate was lower among students who had oral sex exclusively (12% for those who had never had sexual intercourse).

■ SEX AND SUBSTANCE USE

In 2013, 24% of students who had ever had sexual intercourse reported using alcohol or other substances before they had sex the last time. The rate reflected a decline from 32% five years earlier.

And just in case you're wondering, McCreary Centre Society and other researchers have found no evidence that youth will be influenced to try a risky behaviour if they're asked a question about it. So we don't need to worry that simply asking preteens or teens a survey question will plant an idea that they will then act upon.

Before we go further, I think it's worth clearing up some misconceptions about pregnancy. I find that Grade 6 and 7 students have lots of questions and even more misinformation about how it happens and how it doesn't. It's hard to believe, but those old tales and wild rumours we heard growing up about what will prevent pregnancy are still alive and well to a certain extent. In case you've forgotten, let me remind you what some of these are.
- ■ If you stand up and have sex the sperm will fall out.
- ■ If you have sex in a hot tub or lake, the water will wash the sperm out.
- ■ If a woman urinates after sex, the sperm will come out too (as if women urinate out of their vaginas).

- You can't get pregnant the first time you have sex, you can't get pregnant during your period, and the list goes on.

Of course, none of the above is true! At the very least, discussing the ridiculousness of these myths can give you and your preteen a good laugh. But remember to approach the conversation in a general way – "Do you think many teens today believe these myths?" "Where do they get this misinformation?" – so that your child feels like you see them as the expert rather than a misinformed youth.

Talking about unplanned pregnancy (or any sexual health topic for that matter) is easiest when you can use a TV show, movie, article, or relevant real-life situation as the conversation-starter. Remember the movie *Juno* starring the incredibly talented Canadian actor Ellen Page? That movie is a two-hour long teachable moment! After watching it together, you could ask your preteen these questions.

> Is it true that you can have a baby when your 12-14

- How did Juno's unplanned pregnancy affect her life?
- How would her experience have been different if she hadn't had the support of her parents?
- How did her peers react to her pregnancy?
- What were her options?
- What made her decision easy or difficult?
- How did her pregnancy affect her relationship?
- Are partners always supportive?
- What if they want different things?
- How would a teenager support a child financially?
- How would a teenager finish school when they are pregnant or parenting?
- How did Juno's pregnancy affect her day-to-day life?
- How would a pregnancy affect a person's long-term plans and goals?
- How was Juno's pregnancy portrayed in the same way as or differently than on reality shows?

Juno is just one of countless movies or TV shows that could be used to start a conversation about unplanned pregnancy. If you're looking for an example of what teenage pregnancy and parenting *are not*, ask your child to suggest a reality show for you to watch together. No one said using teachable moments would be painless!

I want to acknowledge that not all teen pregnancies are destined for disaster. In my role as a family support worker years ago, with pregnant and parenting teens, many of the young people I worked with were excellent parents and were able to raise their children in healthy, loving, stable environments. Several were single parents, and most had little or no family support. It wasn't easy for them and they made lots of sacrifices, but they were great parents – better parents than some adults I've come across in my work. We need to share these success stories with our preteens as well, to make sure we don't perpetuate the stereotype that teen parents are incompetent or, even worse, failures.

Along these lines, I suggest you reassure your preteen that if, in the future, they or their partner were ever to face an unplanned pregnancy, they can tell you about it and that you will support them in any way you can. Gulp.

Although I don't think it's necessary before high school to teach the ins and outs of all contraceptive methods, it's worth letting your preteen know about the proper use of condoms and the availability of emergency contraception (EC). Take a deep breath; this is just information they can put in their back pocket for later! Remember, the key is to say a bit more than we think we need to, a bit sooner than we think need to.

By now, preteens should have a general idea of how condoms work and how they're used. But here are some extra bits of information that reflect the most common questions Grade 6 and 7 students ask me.

- They're disposable, so they should only be used once.
- They have an expiry date. When used after they've expired, condoms are less effective (heat breaks down latex).
- There are two types of condoms: novelty condoms and condoms meant to prevent pregnancy and the spread of infection. Don't use a novelty condom for anything but fun.
- Buy condoms at a reputable drugstore or grocery store, not from airport or restaurant bathroom dispensers or novelty shops.

Using a condom properly takes practice. It's a good idea to practice putting a condom on yourself (or on your partner) a few times, following the directions carefully, before using it for real.

If they work properly (which they usually do), condoms are very effective at preventing pregnancy, as well as STIs passed through the exchange of bodily fluids. They *do not* protect against STIs passed through skin-to-skin contact.

Unlike other forms of contraception, emergency contraception (EC) can be used *after* intercourse to prevent pregnancy. But as its name suggests, it's for emergencies only. EC is not something to use on a regular basis, but it is a simple and safe way to prevent pregnancy, if needed. There are two hormonal types of emergency contraception pills available in Canada: progestin-only pills (Plan B), and combined estrogen and progestin pills (Yuzpe regimen). In both methods, the sooner the pills are taken the more effective they are, but they *can* be taken up to 120 hours (5 days) after unprotected vaginal intercourse, when a contraceptive method fails, or after a sexual assault.

In addition to being available from your doctor, from walk-in or youth clinics, and from hospital emergency department, EC is now available in Canadian pharmacies without a prescription (regardless of age). The cost varies depending on which EC is used and where it's purchased. Emergency contraception can also be bought in advance and stored for use at a later time.

TALKING ABOUT STIs

According to the 2013 BC Adolescent Health Survey, 3% of students who had had sexual intercourse reported an STI, which was lower than in 2008 and 2003 (4%). This is a step in the right direction, but preteens have also heard tons of misinformation about STIs and we need to clear this up for them. For example, they may get the impression through media and gossip that only people who "sleep around" get STIs. Yes, the more sexual partners you have, the greater the chance you'll be exposed to an infection. That's basic math. But someone can get an STI the first time they have sexual contact of any kind. And someone who's had only one sexual partner could have an STI.

I've also heard students mistakenly assume that once you treat an STI, it's gone for life. But just because you've had, say, chlamydia once doesn't mean you won't ever get it again. And if you have it, your partner needs to be treated for it as well, so the infection doesn't get passed back and forth.

Other STI myths centre around how they can and cannot be transmitted. From time to time, I get questions asking if it's possible to get an STI from a toilet seat. I'm happy to report that the chances are slim to none. Many kids believe that you can only get an STI from vaginal or anal sex, but they need to know that *any* sexual activity involving skin-to-skin genital contact (even digital sex), or the exchange of bodily fluids (such as oral sex) can transmit an infection. And, believe it or not, even some high school students are surprised to hear that oral contraception ("The Pill") offers no protection against STIs.

When it comes to STIs, I find Grade 6 and 7 students mostly have questions about transmission. But when they ask, "How are STIs spread from person to person?" what they're really asking is, "Can I get one and how do I make sure I don't?" The answer is, "by keeping your genitals to yourself!" Sometimes they ask me detailed questions like, "What do herpes look like?" but more often they're interested in the bigger picture of prevention and transmission, which is what I find more useful to focus on.

NOT-SO-FUN FACTS:

HPV is one of the most common sexually-transmitted infections (STIs), with more than 75% of Canadians estimated to have at least one HPV infection in their lifetime. There are over 100 types of HPV, including more than 40 types that involve the genitals. Up to ten of the HPV subtypes have been linked to various cancers (cervix, throat, tongue, anus, penis, and vulva).

Students agree with me that open communication and honesty are key to a healthy relationship, and that partners should discuss their health history before having sex of any kind. But because someone may be too embarrassed to be honest, and because some STIs don't have any symptoms, getting tested is crucial. If a young person doesn't feel comfortable going to their family doctor to get tested for STIs, they can go to a sexual health or youth clinic, a walk-in medical clinic, or a designated STI testing centre in their community. Here, where I am in British Columbia, an Options for Sexual Health clinic is a great choice for teens (and people of all ages).

When discussing testing with preteens and teens I ask them, "Would it be fair to ask your partner to get tested if you aren't willing to go yourself?" (obviously, no) and "What if someone doesn't want to get tested, what could that mean?" They respond quickly with a resounding, "Maybe they're hiding something!" I explain that, more realistically, hesitance to get tested could be an indication of not being ready (or mature enough or comfortable enough or responsible enough) for a sexual relationship. Which is okay too!

Grade 6 and 7 kids often express fear around the actual experience of STI testing. Let your preteen know that, for the most part, it's painless. Some tests require a blood sample, some need a urine sample, and others (like HPV) can be tested for during a regular Pap smear.

We can never remind our kids too often that getting an STI isn't a death sentence. Yes, some STIs are more serious than others. Some can cause infertility. But the STIs that are bacterial infections – such as chlamydia, gonorrhea, and syphilis – can be treated (if caught early) with antibiotics. Having an STI also doesn't mean you can never have sex again. It just requires open communication with partners and your doctor to prevent transmission. I don't mean to downplay the impact that an STI can have on a person's life and their relationships, but we need to get rid of the stigma that still exists around these infections. This stigma also prevents some people from being tested and treated. And although we don't have a cure for viral infections, there are medications that can control symptoms of the infection, or slow its progression. We also have vaccines for hepatitis B and HPV.

◼ HPV

Most parents have heard about the HPV (human papilloma virus) vaccination program for Grade 6 girls here in Canada but have lots of questions about what HPV is, how serious HPV is, and whether HPV vaccines are safe. Here are the basics.

In most cases, HPV infections are asymptomatic and clear on their own within 6–12 months. Some types of HPV cause skin and genital warts that may require treatment. HPV is a ubiquitous virus found on the skin and genitals and is easily passed from one person to another.

Luckily, two HPV vaccines are approved for use in Canada: Cervarix and Gardasil. These vaccines offer good protection against several types of HPV and are most effective when given between the ages of 9 and 26, with the idea of vaccinating a person *before* sexual contact with others. Gardasil protects against four HPV subtypes: the two that cause the majority of HPV-related cancers (HPV-16 and 18) as well as the two that cause the majority of skin and genital warts (HPV-6 and 11). Gardasil is currently being offered free of charge through a vaccination program for Grade 6 girls in Canadian schools in an effort to reduce the rates of HPV infections that lead to cervical and other cancers.

Because of its link to oral and other genital cancers, HPV vaccines have also been approved in Canada for use on boys and men. But it's expensive (at the time of this writing, a full course of the vaccine costs up to $500) and currently only the provinces of Alberta, Manitoba, Nova Scotia, Prince Edward Island, and Quebec have extended the school-based vaccination program to boys. British Columbia is being encouraged to do the same.

There's been a step in the right direction, with BC's Ministry of Health recently announcing that at-risk boys and young men who have sex with men (MSM) can arrange for the HPV immunization free of charge by visiting their local public health unit. This program will also be delivered through specialized clinics and for street-involved youth. Making Gardasil more accessible to the MSM population is important, because they're at increased risk for HPV-related oral, anal, and penile cancers. Since boys and young men are unlikely to self-identify as MSM before their first sexual relationship, the vaccine's benefit is greatest when given well before an adolescent becomes sexually active.

How safe are HPV vaccines? Vaccines are only approved for use in Canada if they're proven to be safe and effective. Since this HPV vaccine was approved, 175 million doses have been provided worldwide. Ongoing monitoring of the vaccine shows it continues to be safe and effective at preventing infections and cancers caused by HPV.

■ TESTICULAR HEALTH

The Canadian Cancer Society reports that testicular cancer is the most common cancer in young men 15–29 years of age. The incidence is lowest before puberty, increases significantly after age 14, peaks around age 30, and declines by age 60. While we're still trying to understand the causes of and risk factors associated with this type of cancer, we need to talk to our kids about it in a way that's preventative and non-threatening. It's all part of teaching them to take responsibility for their health as they get older.

The good news is that, if caught early, testicular cancer has a very high cure rate. But it spreads fast and even a week can make a difference. I encourage Grade 6 and 7 boys to get in the habit of examining their testicles on a regular basis. I explain that if I had testicles I would examine them once a week, maybe on "Testicle Tuesdays"? I'm a bit of a keener when it comes to my health, though, so it would be great if they could do a check even just once a month.

Once the roaring laughter subsides, I explain that in the bath or the shower is the best place to do a testicular exam, because when the skin is wet it's easiest to feel possible lumps. All they have to do is put their fingers over each testicle and feel under the skin (scrotum) for any lumps or bumps. They're also looking for any change in the texture of the scrotum, pain, or redness or swelling (often the first sign). If they notice anything different than the last time, I instruct them to tell a parent right away and they'll probably make an appointment to see the doctor. Meg used to always joke that boys don't need to bring the whole family into the bathroom to have a look. Just telling one parent would be fine.

More good news: nine times out of ten, a lump will have nothing to do with cancer. It could be a cyst or a fibroid – nothing to worry about. But I explain to students that it's better to have it looked at so they don't stress out for no reason. And again, most testicular cancers can be cured if caught early. It's important to note here that it's normal for one testicle to hang lower than the other and that one is bigger than the other.

Of course, we don't want to instill paranoia or fear in our kids unnecessarily, but this is an example of a good habit we can teach early. By the way, I don't teach kids to do breast self-exams at this age because their breasts are still growing and will be lumpy and bumpy until the end of high school (or so) when the breasts stop growing. We don't want them to confuse these healthy *nodes* with a tumour. Having said that, I am a huge fan of young people knowing what their bodies look and feel like and reporting any differences they notice to a parent. As adults, I urge women to do regular breast self-exams, but more on that later.

TIPS FOR TALKING TO INTERMEDIATES (GRADES 4–7)

Acknowledge discomfort. You could say, **"I remember feeling super grossed out about sex growing up, so I don't blame you for feeling the same way. But this is important stuff that will help you make smart decisions about your body and I know you're mature enough to handle it. I'll always be here to talk with you about anything."**

Explore educational websites and YouTube clips or do another activity together while chatting. Sitting side-by-side is often more comfortable for intermediates (as opposed to staring at an adult in the face while talking about freaky topics).

Get books from the library or bookstore and leave them around the house – on the coffee table, beside the toilet, on their bed, in the bookshelf. I promise they'll read them when their friends are over. Read the books first so you can use specifics as conversation starters, and let them know that you'll check in later in the week to see if they have questions.

Pause the PVR when watching TV together to explain or comment on a relevant storyline or commercial. This is why PVRs were invented!

While driving, share about a news story or Facebook post you came across. Even a three-minute conversation is valuable. Plus, they can't escape a moving car.

Leave juicy sexual health articles on the breakfast table and ask that your intermediate read them as they are eating. Discuss them later during a hot chocolate date or on the way to school.

Ask general questions that position your intermediate as the expert *and* that give information: **"A study came out this week reporting that most teens aren't having sex. Does that surprise you?"** Kids love it when adults ask them about grown-up stuff.

Nothing replaces face-to-face conversations, but texting a link to an article could lead to an interesting exchange.

Remember that you don't need to know everything about sex, just have resources handy (for example, **www.urbandictionary.com**). If they ask you a question that stumps you, say **"Let's find out together!"** or **"Good question. Can I get back to you on that?"**

Make sure some of your alone time together doesn't have a discussion agenda. Otherwise, they'll start to dread hanging out with you.

Recruit close friends and family members your child sees as allies. They can help you tick off your list of important conversations, as opportunities arise. Don't take it personally, but sometimes allies have better luck engaging intermediates because they don't see it as "Mom going off again." Sleepovers for my stepdaughters at my sister's place have always been not only fun, but secretly educational too, especially when the girls were younger!

▰ INTERMEDIATE CHECKLIST (GRADES 6-7)

Your Grade 6 or 7 child should know everything the previous age groups have learned, plus

- smart decision-making regarding social media, including discussion of cyberbullying, sexting, and selfies
- how to think critically about pornography
- more about sexual consent in the context of relationships
- how to think critically about gender stereotypes
- what makes for a healthy relationship
- factors to consider when exploring emotional readiness for a sexual relationship
- the different types of sexual activity and possible physical outcomes: STIs (myths, transmission, prevention, testing, and treatment) and pregnancy
- that most teens are not sexually active
- about condoms and emergency contraception (EC) use
- the importance of taking responsibility of one's health (for example, testicular self-examinations)

RESOURCES

FOR PARENTS

WEBSITES
- http://www.mcs.bc.ca/pdf/From_Hastings_Street_To_Haida_Gwaii.pdf – BC Adolescent Health Survey, McCreary Centre Society (2013)
- www.smartsexresource.com – BC Centre for Disease Control
- www.cancer.ca – Canadian Cancer Society.
- www.cancer.org – American Cancer Society
- www.optbc.org – Options for Sexual Health
- http://www.sexualityandu.ca – Society of Obstetricians and Gynaecologists of Canada (SOGC)
- www.urbandictionary.com

ARTICLE
- "HPV and Oral Cancers: Making The Case For Broader Vaccinations," by Allan Hovan, in *The Bridge* (Nov/Dec 2014).

FOR INTERMEDIATE CHILDREN

EMPOWERMENT WEBSITES
- www.gurl.com
- www.newmoon.org
- www.solegirls.org
- www.safeteen.ca
- www.discoverygirls.com
- www.beinggirl.com
- www.boyslife.com
- www.pinkshirtday.ca
- www.goodmenproject.com
- www.amysmartgirls.com

BOOKS ON EMPOWERMENT AND SEXUAL HEALTH

- *All Made Up: A Girl's Guide to Seeing through Celebrity Hype and Celebrating Real Beauty*, by Audrey D. Brashich.
- *Am I Weird or Is This Normal?: Advice and Info to Get Teens in the Know* by Marlin S. Potash and Laura Potash Fruitman.
- *It's Perfectly Normal: Changing Bodies, Growing Up, Sex, and Sexual Health* and *It's So Amazing!: A Book about Eggs, Sperm, Birth, Babies, and Families* by Robie H. Harris.
- *My Body, Myself for Boys* and *My Body, Myself for Girls*, by Lynda and Area Madaras.
- *Puberty Boy*, by Geoff Price.
- *Puberty Girl*, by Shushann Movsessian.
- *Stick Up for Yourself! Every Kid's Guide to Personal Power and Positive Self-Esteem*, by L. Raphael and G. Kaufman.
- *The Body Book for Boys*, by Grace Norwich.
- *The Boy's Body Book: Everything You Need to Know for Growing Up You*, by Kelli Dunham.
- *The Care and Keeping of You: The Body Book for Younger Girls*, and other books in the American Girl series for girls aged eight and up. (These books offer valuable support and guidance on a range of emotional and academic issues associated with growing up.)
- *The Looks Book: A Whole New Approach to Beauty, Body Image, and Style*, by the creators of www.gurl.com.
- *What's Happening to Me?*, by Peter Mayle.
- *What's Happening to Me?* (boys), by Alex Frith.
- *What's Happening to Me?* (girls), by Sue Meredith.

BOOKS ON RELATIONSHIPS

- *A Smart Girl's Guide: Boys*, by Nancy Holyoke (American Girl Library)
- *Drama*, by Raina Telgemeier.
- *Flipped*, by Wendelin Van Draanen.
- *Stargirl*, by Jerry Spinelli.

MAGAZINES FOR GIRLS

- *American Girl*, ages 7 and up www.americangirl.com
- *Discovery Girls*, ages 8 and up www.discoverygirls.com
- *New Moon*, ages 8 and up, www.newmoon.org
- *Vervegirl*, ages 13 and up, www.vervegirl.com

10. Relationships and Healthy Boundaries

10. Relationships and Healthy Boundaries

ADOLESCENTS (GRADES 8–12)

JOY AND PAIN, SUNSHINE AND RAIN

Okay, bonus points for parents who are humming the awesome '90s rap song by Rob Base & DJ E-Z Rock right now. Doesn't its title describe high school romance perfectly?

By the time high school rolls around, my guess is that you'll have already started an ongoing conversation about relationships with your teen. You'll have talked about what a healthy relationship looks and feels like, and you'll have discussed general guidelines around dating, based on your family values and beliefs. Hasn't happened? That's okay – baby steps.

Chances are good that teens will experience their first serious relationship sometime during high school, but some won't. Maybe relationships just aren't on their radar yet. Some are questioning their sexual attraction so aren't sure *who* they want to be in a relationship with. (If you know that's the case, let them know that this is normal and do what you can to support them through it.) Others are too busy to manage a relationship, and that's fine too. Whatever the reason, this is perfectly normal. Not having to deal with teen romance is a relief to many parents who are thus spared the drama and heartbreak that often comes with first love! But other parents worry if their teen *isn't* in a relationship. They wonder, for example, if their teen is missing out, or is developmentally delayed, or isn't seen by others as "relationship material." Remember, though, that it's much more socially (and societally) acceptable now to be single than it was when we were growing up. And young people today certainly don't feel rushed to pick a life partner before they hit their 20s!

Regardless of *when* they happen, first serious relationships can be all-consuming, joyous, intense, exhilarating, agonizing, and heartbreaking all at them same time. And although parents' understandable first instinct may be to discourage them, that's the last thing we should do. If our teen senses we disapprove of them being in a relationship, they'll shut down, withhold information, and stop coming to us for support. So questions like, "Don't you think you're a bit young to be in a serious relationship?" are the opposite of productive. Instead, say things like, **"Sounds like you've been hanging out a lot with Maya. She seems like an awesome person."** Or **"I get the feeling that Jason is really special to you. I can't wait to meet him."** Showing support for their relationship demonstrates that you validate their feelings and that's what will keep them coming back to you for guidance and sharing. Because you want to be as involved in their relationship as possible, this is super important. And remember not to assume that your teen's relationship is heterosexual.

Invite their partner over for dinner, include them in family outings and events, ask about them and get to know their family if it looks like the relationship is going to last a while. And, whatever you do, don't introduce them to relatives as your teen's "special friend." That's patronizing. We need to validate their relationship and take it seriously. Of course, embracing your teen's partner and their relationship doesn't mean you need to allow sleepovers every weekend. Most parents wouldn't feel comfortable with that, but go with what feels right to you. You might also want to put some boundaries around where and how they're hanging out in your home. If they want to be in your teen's bedroom together, maybe the door stays open. And they should know that you'll probably peek in to say "Hi!" on your way to the bathroom. A healthy dose of paranoia that you're going to show up unannounced is a foolproof way of keeping their visit PG. I mean, the reality is that they can and probably will do whatever they want when you are out, but this is about respecting your home, especially when others are around.

But what if you think your daughter's boyfriend dresses like a scrub, has the personality of a door handle, and the intelligence of Joey from *Friends*, but isn't as endearing. Well, suck it up. Maybe your daughter will eventually find that out for herself, or maybe not. It's *her* relationship, so you can't make that decision for her. And remember that making disparaging remarks (even jokingly) about her boyfriend could result in her being protective and defensive, which in turn could work against you. The last thing you want is for your daughter to tell her boyfriend what you said and for them to see you as the enemy.

If you have concerns about your teen's happiness in their relationship, though, that *is* worth talking about. Still, we need to be gentle and choose our words wisely. Find a time when you can be alone with your teen without distractions, and share your concerns honestly. Relationship therapist Dr. Laura Berman suggests parents could start by saying, **"I've noticed you haven't been yourself lately, you seem sad and distracted. Anything you want to talk about?"** or **"I know relationships aren't always easy, but I'm here for you if you need to talk."**

If those general statements open a conversation, then you can get more specific. That's when you can say, **"Disagreements in a relationship are normal, but it seems like you and Geoff have been arguing more than normal lately. Does it feel that way to you?"** or **"It seemed like Jessica was being a bit grumpy with you when we were at the beach this weekend. Are things okay between you?"** Always end the conversation on a positive note stressing how deserving your teen is of a healthy, happy relationship. There's no reason for them to settle for less, and you'll always be there to support them. Believe it or not, teens are very capable of being in a healthy relationship. But they have little experience, and a lack of good communication skills sometimes gets in the way, so they need our support.

If you're concerned about your teen's safety or well-being in the relationship, that's a different story altogether and you'll need to be more direct. For example, what if your teen's partner is much older than they are (older than a couple years), or you suspect abuse? As tempting as it is, ordering your teen to break up with their partner will backfire. Instead, calmly explain to your teen why you're deeply concerned. Again, be careful not to bad-mouth their partner; they're probably very protective of them and may see you as the problem. Ask lots of open-ended questions and listen carefully.

Keep your judgments to yourself and don't show anger. Gently stress that while it sounds like there are some great things about their relationship, control, manipulation, extreme jealousy, head games, and violent outbursts are *never* okay. You may have to bite off this conversation one chunk at a time so it's more manageable. Not to mention your teen will probably do everything possible to make a break for it. Be gently persistent. Continually remind them that you're there for them in any way they need you.

If you suspect relationship abuse (girls aged 15–24 are most likely to experience it), talk about it and give your teen the phone numbers and websites of resources in your community. It's also worth suggesting that if they aren't totally comfortable talking to you about this, there are other people in their lives who would be trustworthy allies – perhaps an aunt, older sibling, teacher, or a close family friend. Don't take it personally if they confide in someone else; the goal is to get them help.

Eventually, only when your teen is ready, make a break-up plan together. How will they do it? Definitely not on social media or by text. Will they do it when they're alone with their partner? If they're concerned about their safety, they should have someone else present with them. And continue the conversations well after the breakup. It may take a couple of tries.

When it happens for good, *you* may be doing a happy dance, but for your teen the pain of a first breakup can be excruciating. Here's what *not* to say, whether the relationship was healthy or not.

> why do people make out and then dump the person

- Why are you so upset? You only dated for four months!
- Oh it's okay, honey; you'll be over him in no time.
- I never thought she was right for you anyway.
- There are plenty of fish in the sea!
- I can't believe he broke up with you online. What a jerk!
- You can do better.

Instead, offer kind words of support and understanding and let your teen know that you're there for them if they want to talk. Simple nurturing comments like, **"I don't know much about why Maddie broke up with you, but I can imagine how devastated you must be right now. Do you feel like talking about it?"** or **"I get it if you don't want to talk about it, but just know that my heart is hurting for you and I'm here whenever you need me."**

Or share a personal story to show them you understand. I'll never forget my dad sitting on my bed with me after a particularly difficult breakup in Grade 12. He told me about a relationship he had when he was in high school and about how devastated he was when his girlfriend broke up with him. I don't remember there being a life-changing message in the story, but I remember feeling like he "got it." He listened to me. I felt like he took my heartbreak seriously in that moment, even though internally he was probably thinking that it wasn't worth the weekend I spent sobbing in my bedroom and listening to Sinead O'Conner sing "Nothing Compares."

Then again, sometimes it's best to say nothing at all. Instead, offer a distraction from the pain. Take them and a friend to their favourite frozen yogurt place. Have a Netflix marathon. Let them take a day off school to lick their wounds, but then insist that they get back into their regular routine. Getting support from friends at school and slowly recognizing that life will go on will help them heal. And there will come a day (hopefully sooner rather than later) when they wake up and their ex-partner isn't the first thing that comes to mind. You don't need to tell your teen that this process doesn't change much, even when you're an adult.

■ EARNING FREEDOM, SETTING LIMITS, PUSHING BOUNDARIES

Have you ever heard of the parenting book *Get Out of My Life, but First Could You Drive Me & Cheryl to the Mall?* by Anthony Wolfe? Not only does it offer common sense guidance for parents of teens, but the title sums up the teenage years to a tee. Understandably, our kids demand more privacy, freedom, and privileges as they get older. They also want less micro-managing, fewer texts, and fewer questions from us parents (but keep the rides coming). Some parents are more than happy to make this happen for their teen, and expect little accountability or responsibility in return. These are the "cool" parents who are so busy trying to get their kids to like them that they forget teens still need boundaries and limits. Not to mention respect for our time and energy.

Other parents are so stressed out, tired, and busy trying to balance hectic work and family lives that they're relieved to finally have less hands-on parenting now, especially if they have younger children, too. So they check out. Where their teen is going, what they're doing, what's happening at school, and who they're hanging out with slips under the radar and, fingers crossed, no one gets hurt.

There are also some parents who feel that teens should be allowed complete freedom. These parents figure that their teens will find out soon enough about making mistakes and needing to clean up their own messes. The trouble with this philosophy is that sometimes the messes are too big for a teen to deal with alone – sometimes those situations are even life-threatening. Not to mention that the teens of these parents may take *your* teen down with them.

Conscientious parents are somehow able to find a balance. They understand that teens *do* need more freedom to make their own decisions, but also that their teens need to take responsibility for these decisions and learn from their mistakes. This may include less monitoring of their teen's every move, but these parents *aren't* afraid to set reasonable limits and boundaries. It's give and take. Freedom and privileges aren't something teens are entitled to; they're earned. These parents also understand that parenting isn't a popularity contest. If it were, they would never win. They're still deeply involved in their teen's life, but at more of a distance as their child gets older.

I saw Oprah Winfrey speak when she came to town a few years ago and one thing she said about parenting stuck with me. Talking about the young women from Africa she was raising in her home at the time, she suggested that as our teens near the end of high school our role as parents needs to shift. That is, we go from being their "manager" to their "consultant." Rather than making decisions *for* our teens, whenever possible we need to provide them with the information and skills they need to make their own decisions. It sounds easy enough, except that we weren't hired for the job and the interview is ongoing. And, on some days, the benefits don't seem worth it!

But that's down the road a little bit. Until we graduate to being consultants, how do we manage our teens in a way that keeps them safe, but that also honours their maturity and that teaches them responsibility? And what do we do when our teens push our boundaries (which they *will* do) and break our trust? Teens are experts at pushing boundaries, so let's look at three examples of many.

SLEEPOVER SNEAKINESS

Most of us have great memories of sleepovers with friends growing up. Watching movies till all hours of the night, gorging on instant noodles, debriefing the events at the roller rink earlier that night – sleepovers were good clean fun. We want our teens to experience those fun times as well and, for the most part, we don't give it much thought.

But from time to time, doubt sets in. Are they really doing what they said they were going to do? Are they really where they said they would be? And it's not like we can call a landline to confirm their whereabouts. What if they start at friend's house, but go to a party later? In your teen's mind they aren't lying, because they'll end up there *eventually*, right? What if there's a party where the sleepover is happening? What if the parents are out and they have some guys over to play drinking games? Is this your gut trying to tell you something (um, yes) or are you just being paranoid? Suddenly, sleepovers become an exercise in espionage for parents. And sometimes that's just the way it has to be.

As early as you can (preferably in elementary school), respond to every sleepover request with the same basic questions:

- Who's going?
- What are you going to do?
- Who's going to be home?
- Do you want me to drive you and pick you up? (If your teen says "No," consider it a red flag.)

Then touch base with the parent. If you don't have their number, ask your teen for it. If they push back or list reasons why you can't call them, another red flag. You may hear complaints that you're micro-managing, that you're the only parent who's so anal about sleepovers, and that you don't trust them. Maybe past behaviour has eroded your trust and if so, be honest. But regardless of what *other* parents do, you need to know what the plan is. If the plan *is* to go to a party, then that requires a different level of decision-making (we'll get there in the next section).

If, after talking to the parent, you're comfortable that the sleepover is a good idea, then great. If you're on the fence, talk to friends whose teens may be invited as well. Are they allowing *their* teens to go? But trust your gut. If you really don't feel comfortable, explain *why* to your teen. Maybe having a sleepover at your house is a better option. Or, maybe your teen goes to the friend's house, but you pick them up at curfew. Hopefully, your teen will accept one of these Plan Bs, but if not, stand your ground. Remember, if your teen liked every decision you made, you wouldn't be parenting them properly.

■ PARTY PLANNING 101

Whether it's during a sleepover or not, there's a good chance your teen will go to a party without you knowing about it,

sometime during high school. Not being totally honest or omitting certain information about what they're doing and where they're going is a pretty normal *modus operandi* for teens. Think about it; I doubt *any* of us were *completely* honest with our parents when we were teens! Hopefully, you can manage their safety in these situations by already being in the habit of asking important questions before they go out, checking in with them throughout the night, and having clear expectations in terms of what you're okay with, and what you aren't.

Best-case scenario, your teen will tell you about the party they want to go to (because you've already established open dialogue about stuff like this), which will allow you to make an informed decision. Again, here are the standard questions to ask:

- Where is the party?
- How are you getting to and from it?
- How many people do you think will be there?
- Will there be drinking and/or drugs?
- Who's supervising? (*If there's no adult present, that's a deal breaker.*)
- Can I have their phone number to check in? (If they give excuses, red flag.)

If you're confident that the parent and you are on the same page in terms of what's appropriate for teenagers and how the party will be managed if things get out of hand, then your teen gets to go and everyone's happy. Even when you *do* check in with parents, though, remember that your idea of an appropriate party for teens may be very different from *theirs*. Meg recalls speaking to a parent who learned this early on. Luckily this man's son was smart enough to leave the situation as soon as he started to feel uncomfortable.

The father told Meg that he felt really prepared when his son asked him if he could go to his first high school house party. He asked his son all the standard questions and called the parent to check in and get some details. She assured him that she would be there at all times, that she understood how teens are at parties, and that he had nothing to worry about…she was a child psychologist, after all!

The dad decided to allow his son to go to the party and on the way there he reminded his son of their agreement that he would leave if he felt uncomfortable or unsafe. He gave his son his word that he would come and get him if he texted, and that he wouldn't be mad.

Two hours later, a text came in from his son asking to be picked up around the corner from the party. In the car on the way home, the father asked what happened. His son said, "Dad, it sucked. Everyone was drunk. Some kids were throwing up and being really weird." The father was shocked. "But where was Dr. Jones? She promised she'd be there. Where did the alcohol come from?"

"Oh, Dr. Jones gave everyone wine or beer. She said she knows kids need to experiment; she said it was okay…"

Remember the "cool" parents I mentioned earlier? Dr. Jones is a perfect example. She justified providing minors with alcohol by reasoning that she'd rather have the kids party at her home, to keep them safe, despite it being illegal. She was so concerned about the teens having a good time, she didn't think of how quickly the party could get out of hand. Not to mention the possible legal consequences if anything *had* happened to one of the guests.

Some parents take a similar approach by providing their teen with a small amount of alcohol before they head out to a party. Their reasoning is that by giving their teen some alcohol they'll drink in moderation and won't be tempted to share with other kids, or risk mixing types of alcohol. Although some parents see this approach as harm reduction, the alcohol they're giving their teen will probably be gone before they even get to the party. Meanwhile, their *real* alcohol order has been picked up for them by a friend's older sister and is waiting for them when they get there.

When making the decision about a party, it's also a good idea to check in with the parents of your teen's friends. If they aren't allowing their teens to go, this should influence your decision. There's power in numbers in situations like this. Parents can support each other, exchange opinions, and feel more justified in the decision they've made. And if a group of parents decide together that it's *not* going to happen, their teen's argument that "Everyone else's parents are letting them go!" is a non-starter.

By the way, if your teen is asking to go to an "alcohol-free, drug-free" rave to listen to DJs with 700 of their closest friends in an abandoned warehouse outside of town, please say "No." First, raves are *anything but* alcohol and drug-free. What a joke. As if your teen doesn't know already, remind them that hundreds of people (that they don't know, some much older than they are) will show up to the event already wasted and/or high. Not only that, but many raves aren't legal for minors. The "cool" parent may let their 16-year-old lie about their age to get in, but that's the opposite of cool in my opinion. The only exception to the no-rave rule would be those organized for all ages by reputable organizations (such as community centres). Of course, you'll drop them off and pick them up at a pre-arranged time. Or you can go with them. Not kidding.

I don't recommend that teens have sleepovers after a party. Agree that you'll pick them up at curfew, perhaps slightly extended – that way they know they have to sober up enough to face you at the end of the night. Remember Rosalind Wiseman's recommendation that parents cultivate a healthy dose of paranoia? She notes that the safety of teens staying where the party is being held is tempting, but that just gives them a free pass to get wasted. Plus, even the most responsible chaperones have to go to bed at some point. Your teen won't like this plan and will give you every reason they can think of as to why they should be able to sleep over, and how you're the *only* parent that's not allowing it. That's okay. Hold your ground and know that you're doing the right thing.

What about your teen having a party while you're away? Before you go, think carefully about whether it's a good idea to leave them alone at home. My husband and I recently started allowing my oldest stepdaughter to stay home alone for a few nights, but she's never given us a reason not to trust her. Still, we're clear with our expectations before we go: no parties allowed, but she can have a few friends over who we know and trust. So far, so good. She's really proven to us that she can be trusted at home alone. In fact, the other day when we were walking back to the car after lunch with family, I heard her say to her aunt, "I would never have a party when Dad and Saleema are away; it would so not be worth it. I might as well sign my death certificate." Mission accomplished!

Every teen is different, though, and sometimes baby steps make sense. At least the first time you go away, maybe it's a good idea to have an adult family member or friend stay at your house with them. If you have a pet that requires care, that gives you a valid reason to do this.

If your teen will be alone, be clear that no parties are allowed. If you're comfortable with them having a few friends over, specify who and how many. Remember, though, that thanks to Facebook, "a few" can turn into 50 pretty quickly, even if your teen isn't the one spreading the word. Let neighbours know that you're away and that you don't want parties. They can call you if they see anything suspicious. Like puke in their mailbox.

When I talk about parties with parents, they often ask me, "Okay, so let's say we let our teen go to a party. Are we really going to let them drink? How do we know what's appropriate and what's not?" Here's what a parent might say to their teen about drinking at parties.

"I know you're growing up and have shown me that you deserve more freedom to do things like go to parties. I know that drinking alcohol and sometimes taking drugs happens at these parties, and I certainly hope you never do drugs. I'd prefer that you didn't drink either until you're an adult. Not only is it illegal at your age, but when you're drunk (or high) it's really hard to make smart decisions. Your judgment is clouded, and things that seem like a great idea at the time may not be so great after all.

"But I can't control everything you do and I know it's not realistic to expect you not to drink. So my goal, as your parent, is to arm you with good information and hope that you make the smart choices I know you're capable of making. My priority is to keep you safe (and alive), so I'd like us to agree to the following:

- Use moderation. If you want to drink, limit yourself to one or two. And don't do shots.
- Make sure you eat before and throughout the party.
- Don't mix different kinds of alcohol.
- Don't leave your drink unattended.
- Always have a buddy so you can watch out for each other.
- Don't ever get in a car with someone during or after a party, even if they don't seem like they've been drinking.

- Don't trust that "cool" parents are making responsible decisions.
- And if you feel uncomfortable or unsafe, text me. I'll come and get you and I promise I won't be mad.

Believe it or not, teens often tell me that they're secretly glad that their parents have firm rules and guidelines, or that they wish their parents had *more* of them. Rules give teens an "out," a reason *not* to do something they're not comfortable doing. For example, "There's no way I can have another drink; my mom will be here to pick me up in half an hour," or "My dad would kill me if I got in a car after drinking."

We also need to teach teens to trust their gut. I encourage them to pay attention to their bodies, because sometimes physical symptoms will warn them that they're in danger before their head will. If they feel nauseous, get stomach cramps, or have to go to the bathroom, this may be their body telling them to do whatever they can to get out of that situation. In a perfect world, teens would simply be able to say, "I'm not comfortable doing this. Later, losers!" But think about how tough that can be. No one wants to look like a "wuss" or a "goodie-goodie." (Remember that word?! Love it.)

I also encourage parents to say something like, **"Some really dangerous situations, like when you realize the person driving you has been drinking, require more immediate action. That's when it's okay to say, 'Oh, oh. I don't feel good. I think I'm gonna throw up,' or 'I think I just got my period all over your seat. Can you pull over?' Trust me, they will."**

▪ DRESS

Truth time. This has been, hands down, the toughest section of this book to write. For the first time in this whole process of writing, I'm finding that what I want to suggest as an educator isn't consistent with what I do as a parent. Don't judge!

As an educator, I want to tell you that what girls and women wear has *nothing* to do with being harassed or assaulted. We need to start teaching *men* not to harass and assault, and stop teaching women that they're somehow responsible for what happens to them. Enough with the message that women shouldn't dress a certain way, or do certain things so that they don't get raped. I also feel strongly that we, as women, should never have to be concerned with how our appearance might be "distracting" or even "offensive" to others. And I know that we women aren't to blame for this – rape culture is.

I want my girls to be able to express their style and sexuality in any way that feels right for them. I never want them to feel that they have to hide their bodies, especially if it's because they're supposedly "distracting" to others. And I certainly don't want them to worry about what someone else thinks of them because of how they dress. I want them to own their bodies, love their bodies, be proud of them, and feel confident in them. *But…*

Every time I go back-to-school shopping with my stepdaughters, every time they head out for a night with friends, and every day when they head off to school, I ask myself that nasty question, "Is what they're wearing appropriate?" I never knew or even suspected how much I would grow to hate that word, *appropriate*. And if what they're wearing is *inappropriate* in my view, I ask them to change.

I know that our clothing and general appearance send messages to others that may *not* reflect who we truly are. But girls are taught from day one in our hypersexualized society that they have to dress in a revealing, provocative, sexy, adult way to be popular, get noticed, or be seen as girlfriend material. And for many of them, this is the goal. Every day they consume media images, see advertising, listen to music, and interact on social media with their peers, all of which perpetuate the notion that girls and women are valued predominantly for their sexiness. In fact, sexualized clothing for kids, preteens, and teens has become so pervasive that young people don't notice it. Even many parents don't notice it.

I also know that people make judgments about girls based on their clothing: what they're into sexually, what they're not into sexually, and how sexually experienced they are. This could result in my girls getting attention that they don't want and/or aren't equipped to deal with.

Plus, why should everyone who walks by them get to see their bodies? Shouldn't my girls get to choose? But do they really understand yet what it means to share their body in that way, with people they don't even know?

I firmly believe that clothing that's appropriate to wear at the beach would not be appropriate to wear to school, or to a job interview, which is why I generally support reasonable school dress guidelines *for all students*. We need to teach our kids to make good decisions about how they dress. This has nothing to do with whether a person is dressing in a way that's sexy or revealing; it's about respecting the different environments we live in and what's appropriate in each of these settings. But we also have to have the conversation with our kids about *why* these dress codes exist, and about why they're important. And there needs to be freedom within the dress code for them to express their individuality and style in other ways (for example, hair styles and colour, jewellery and other accessories).

We also need to be flexible. Maybe it's not your first choice for your son to walk around the mall with his underwear sticking out the top of his shorts, or for your daughter to go from the beach to the snack bar without a cover-up on. But remember about choosing your battles? Allowing some leeway, especially on weekends or during the summer, will make your life easier. I've definitely learned the value of this as a parent, although it hasn't been easy. I've not always been thrilled with some of my stepdaughters' outfit choices, but I've expanded what I can live with over the years.

That said, we've still drawn some lines we're not willing to let them cross. For example, any clothing that promotes alcohol, homo/transphobia, or sexism is a no-go in our house. Today's clothing trends don't help, either. If you've tried recently to shop for a pair of shorts that don't give a peek-a-boo view of your daughter's buttocks, you feel my pain. And before we're quick to judge the parents of daughters who wear short shorts and crop tops, keep in mind they probably don't know. Chances are their daughter has changed after leaving the house, or keeps a stash of clothes at a friend's house.

In conclusion, let me say that there are no easy answers when it comes to how your teen dresses. You know them best, and you know what feels right to you. Talk to your teen about your concerns, be flexible where you can, and trust your gut. What I *do* know is that how girls and women dress will continue to be an issue until we no longer live in a rape culture. Until then, girls and women will have to think twice about what they're wearing.

■ RESOURCES

FOR PARENTS

WEBSITES AND ARTICLES

■ www.safeteen.ca (a website for workshops that teach powerful alternatives to violence)

■ http://raisingchildren.net.au/relationships/teen_relationships.html (a website featuring articles about teenage romance, relationships and intimacy, etc.)

■ https://www.psychologytoday.com/blog/sticky-bonds/200906/teenagers-in-love (an article about parents' reactions to teen romance)

BOOKS

■ *Get Out of My Life, but First Could You Drive Me & Cheryl to the Mall?: A Parent's Guide to the New Teenager*, by Anthony Wolfe.

■ *Queen Bees and Wannabes: Helping Your Daughter Survive Cliques, Gossip, Boyfriends, and the New Realities of Girl World*, by Rosalind Wiseman.

■ *Talking to Your Kids about Sex: Turning "The Talk" into a Conversation for Life*, by Dr. Laura Berman.

FOR TEENS

WEBSITES

■ www.scarleteen.com
■ www.kidshealth.org
■ www.stayteen.org

BOOKS

■ *Changing Bodies, Changing Lives: A Book for Teens on Sex and Relationships*, by Ruth Bell.

- *Chicken Soup for the Soul: Teens Talk Relationships*, by Jack Canfield.
- *Don't Sweat the Small Stuff for Teens: Simple Ways to Keep Your Cool in Stressful Times*, by Richard Carlson.
- *Girls and Sex: Navigating the Complicated New Landscape*, by Peggy Orenstein.
- *In Love and in Danger: A Teen's Guide for Breaking Free of Abusive Relationships*, by Barrie Levy.
- *S.E.X., second edition: The All-You-Need-To-Know Sexuality Guide to Get You Through Your Teens and Twenties*, by Heather Corinna.
- *The 7 Habits of Highly Effective Teens: Revised and Updated Edition*, by Sean Covey.
- *Yes Your Parents Are Crazy!: A Teen Survival Guide*, by Michael J. Bradley.

ARTICLES

- http://www.huffingtonpost.com/news/teen-relationships/ (a link to a series of articles written for teens on relationships)

11. Sex Talk? No Sweat.

11. Sex Talk? No Sweat.

■ ADOLESCENTS (GRADES 8–12)

■ SMART DECISIONS START HERE

Traditionally, sex education in high schools has been fear-based and problem-focused. Curricula have taken a "Watch out!" alarmist approach, with students being warned that getting pregnant will ruin their lives and that getting an STI can kill them. Not only does this approach not work, but it's doing our teens a huge disservice. It also characterizes sex as wrought with nightmare consequences, and ignores the fact that a sexual relationship is usually a positive thing in a person's life.

It's easy to blame teachers, but the reality is that they aren't properly supported in teaching sex education. They often aren't given adequate training or up-to-date resources, and some just aren't comfortable teaching the subject. We need do better if we expect teachers to teach our children about sexual health in a meaningful way. As it stands, our expectations are unfair.

As a result, the task of teaching our teens about sex and sexuality falls to us parents. Some parents, not surprisingly, are afraid to address sex in a positive way for fear that if we make sex sound too good, every teen will be doing it ten times a week. Not true. Within the context of giving life-saving safety information, we need to emphasize at every opportunity that sex is a good thing. Between two consenting adults in a healthy, respectful relationship, sex is great. It's a way that people not only reproduce but, more commonly, a way that people show their love and affection for one another. And *it feels good*, people! If we don't acknowledge this, our teens will catch on that we're not telling the whole story and we'll lose credibility.

Being sex positive also includes recognizing that teens' sexual feelings are real and that they're powerful. One way we can show our teens that we understand this is by talking more about masturbation as a healthy, safe way to satisfy their natural sexual urges. Share with your teen that we know from research that most people in the world, at every age, masturbate. As Meg says, "If God didn't want us to masturbate, our

> *[handwritten note: On average, how many times are you supposed to Masterbute in a month?]*

arms would be shorter!" Some parents take their daughter to buy a vibrator to enhance masturbation. I'm not suggesting you have to run to your nearest sex shop to make the purchase, but do what feels right to you. And if your teens share a room, make sure they each have some private time in there. Let's teach our teens to embrace their sexual feelings in a healthy way. Let's also teach them that they don't need to rely on someone else to give them sexual pleasure. In fact, sex will be even better when the time comes if they masturbate, because they already know their body and what makes them feel good.

When it comes to having sex with another person, remember that many teens aren't (and never will be) interested in vaginal sex, because they identify as gay, or they're just not attracted to vaginas. Some teens are exploring their sexual attraction and haven't yet decided who they want to share their sexuality with, and that's just fine, too. Knowing this, conversations need to include all kinds of sex and relationships, and pregnancy as an outcome (positive or negative) shouldn't be the only focus. Having said that, research shows that youth who are "questioning" their sexuality are actually more likely than "straight" youth to face an unplanned pregnancy. Counterintuitive, I know, but when sex with someone of the opposite sex is unplanned or happens outside of a relationship, contraception is less likely to be used. This shows us how everyone needs a broad range of information.

We also need to recognize that teen sex doesn't always happen in the context of a committed relationship. They "hook up," they have "friends with benefits," and, particularly in these situations, sex may not be planned. My point is that even if your teen isn't in a relationship right now, the topic of sex is still relevant. We may not have the luxury of guiding our teen through the decision-making process if sex happens spontaneously, or in a context they think we disapprove of.

Something else to consider is that we know from statistics that teens are actually more likely to engage in oral sex than vaginal sex during high school. Although we've come a long way in recent years in terms of helping teens understand that oral sex is "real" sex, many still view it as safer (because there's no risk of pregnancy) and less intimate than vaginal sex. For this reason, it's possible that teens have multiple oral sex partners and, therefore, increased risk of STIs.

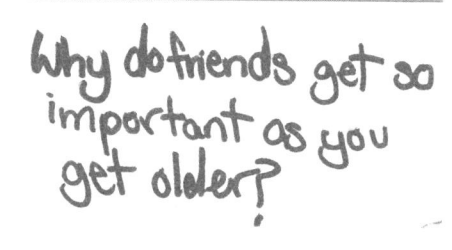

Why do friends get so important as you get older?

It's also important to know that, in heterosexual encounters, girls are usually the givers of oral sex and boys the receivers. And regardless of whether it's inside or outside the context of a relationship, a girl can quickly be branded a slut if word gets around. Talk with your teen about the importance of equality. In a healthy sexual relationship, pleasure is shared. It's not fair to expect someone to do something to your body when you don't feel comfortable doing the same thing to them. Also, teach your teen that it's not cool to kiss and tell. Everyone involved deserves to have their privacy respected.

No conversation with teens about sex would be complete without an appreciation of how powerful peer and societal pressure to be sexually active can be. Girls learn from their peers, media, and our society in general that they should put a good chunk of effort into how they look, mostly so that they can get attention from guys. As a result, they may mistakenly believe that they have to get or respond to this attention with sex, or at least with the promise of sex. Girls are also trying to navigate some pretty impossible mixed messages about their sexuality. On the one hand, they're taught to preserve their sexual purity, but are teased for being "frigid" if they're in a relationship and don't want sex. Even stronger is the message is that if they want to stay in the game they need to "give it up." Again, this comes with the risk of being branded as a slut, especially if sex happens outside of a committed relationship.

Boys, on the other hand, are taught that if they aren't sexually experienced at a young age something's wrong with them. They brag about their sexual conquests (even if they're imaginary) to gain approval, and to be seen as a "pimp" or "player" by their friends. Years ago, after a session teaching a class of Grade 10 students, one of the boys disclosed to me that he had been at a house party the weekend before, and one of the girls there had offered to perform oral sex on him in one of the back bedrooms. He barely knew her and (like most teenage boys) wasn't interested in the least, so politely said, "Nah, I'm good," and walked back to his group of friends. He then made the mistake of telling them what had just happened. When they found out that he refused oral sex from a "hot chick," they teased him for days about being a wuss and a fag. I worried about what this boy would do the next time someone gave him a similar offer. Would he say, "Yah, sure," to avoid being harassed again by his friends?

Talk about this double standard with your teen, and remind them that good friends and partners respect each other's decisions. Ask questions, but be careful to keep them general: **"Do you think people your age feel pressure to have sex?" "Are pressures to have sex different for boys and girls? How so?" "Why is it socially acceptable for boys to be sexually experienced, but not for girls?"** and **"Do you think many people have sex during high school?"** Position them as the expert, teens love it when they're given the opportunity to teach their parent something. And if you feel comfortable, share your experience of peer pressure and the sexual double standard when *you* were in high school. Have things changed since then?

Obviously, you can't make sexual decisions for your teen (although life would be a lot easier if you could! Or so we tell ourselves). Best-case scenario, we can be involved in their decision-making by being an objective sounding board, sharing our experience when appropriate, and offering scientific information. It also doesn't hurt to let your teen know that you've never heard an adult say, "Gee, I wish I started having sex earlier!"

Seriously, though, don't be afraid to offer your teen tips on how to make any decision that involves their body. Talk about how their head, their heart, and their physical body need to be aligned in order to truly give sexual consent. Only when that happens will sex be the best it can be, which is what you hope for them.

If your teen shares with you that they're feeling pressure from their partner to have sex and they're certain they're not ready to go there, take their openness as a compliment. Be grateful that they trust you as a support and praise them profusely for their courage to share. This is a good time to revisit the concept of sexual consent. Let your teen know that it's okay to say "no" and that their partner needs to respect this, even if they're disappointed or don't understand. It's not your teen's job to justify why they don't want to have sex. And if not having sex is a deal breaker for their partner, well, better the relationship ends now than later. Sounds simple, and I know it's not. But we need to help our teens understand that no relationship is worth compromising our own personal boundaries and values. Not only that, but someone in a healthy relationship would never want their partner to do this.

> 1. What can you do if you love/like someone but isn't ready to have sex and you don't want to send the wrong impression

Brainstorm and practice some specific phrases using what's known as the "sandwich technique," which involves placing a statement that may be perceived as negative or disappointing to the other person between two positive or affirming statements. For example, your teen could say to their partner, **"I love that we're getting closer, and I'm not ready to have sex. I also love that I can be honest with you about how I'm feeling,"** or **"I care so much about you that I want to be really sure I'm ready to have sex. I'm not ready right now and I'm glad we're getting closer in other ways."**

Of course, some teens aren't as affected by pressure from others and decide whether or not to have sex for reasons of their own. This is the time to ask lots of questions about what's factoring into their decision, especially if they've decided to have sex. Do they want to take their relationship to that next level of intimacy? Maybe they need some ideas for how they can do this without having sex. Is their body telling them they're ready? If it's sexual arousal that's the driving force, remind them that they can satisfy these natural feelings on their own. At that point they may blow you off, but at least you've planted the seed. And congratulations on getting that far!

An equally important question is, "Is your *partner* ready for sex?" Remind your teen that silence doesn't indicate consent. The only real way a person can let you know they're ready for a sexual relationship is for them to tell you using words. It's not enough for them to *act* like they're okay with it. At the same time, we all need to watch our partner's non-verbal cues. If they're pulling away, look physically uncomfortable or seem hesitant, they're trying to tell us something. As sexual activity progresses, your teen needs to check in with their partner every now and then with simple questions like, **"Are you okay with this?" "Are you having fun?" "Would you like me to…?"** It's never okay to be pushy or to make a partner feel bad for saying no. And remind your teen that if their partner consents and then changes their mind, that's fine too. Consenting once doesn't mean they have to consent later; each person is always free to reconsider what they do or do not consent to. And if their partner is drunk, passed out, or sleeping, it's game off.

The bottom line is that having sex with someone who doesn't consent is not only *not* sexy, it's assault. Sex is best when both partners are 100% ready, on board, and feel respected by their partner.

Most parents aren't thrilled when their teen becomes sexually active, and being positive can be difficult. As hard as it is, though, we need to give our teens space to make their own decisions about their body. We can give information, we can support them in their decision-making process, but at the end of the day the decision is theirs to make. Stay involved and interested, continue to offer information and guidance, and trust that your teen is armed to make smart decisions when it comes to sex. Tell them, **"I know you're old enough and mature enough to make your own decisions about your body, and I trust you'll do what's right for you. Even though I may not always agree, I respect your decisions and will always be here to support you without judging you or getting mad."

While supporting your teen as they navigate decisions around their sexuality, it's also important to make sure they have the scientific information they need to make smart decisions and stay healthy. Besides providing practical information, discussing the not-so-great aspects of sex, like STIs or unplanned pregnancy, sends the message to your teen that you're here for them should one of these outcomes happen. It also counteracts the romanticized, unrealistic view of sex they see in movies and online, where nothing ever goes wrong. In a perfect world, parents would have already started an ongoing conversation about preventing STIs, so now's the time to give them a refresher.

▰ SORTING OUT STI MYTHS

Outlining each one of these in detail would make this feel too much like a medical textbook, so I'm going to talk about STIs in a more general way. This is the approach I take with teens in the classroom as well. Believe it or not, some of the same myths about STIs we heard growing up are still circulating among teens. I suggest you break them down for your teen one by one. Maybe during a game of True or False over dinner? Or using the old, **"I heard on the radio today that a lot of teens still think you can't get an STI from oral sex. Is that true?"** trick. Here are 11 myths teens have asked me about lately.

Only people who sleep around get STIs

STIs don't discriminate. They don't care where you live, how much money you have, how many times a day you shower, how often you have sex, or who you have sex with. Anyone can get one, even the first time you have sexual contact with someone.

Remind your teen not to jump to the conclusion that their partner has been sleeping around if they test positive for an STI. The part-

TALK SEX TODAY

FUN FACT:
We know of over 50 STIs, with 8 of them being the most common ones that people recognize: HIV/AIDS, hepatitis B, hepatitis C, HPV (human papilloma virus), chlamydia, gonorrhea, herpes and syphilis.

ner may have contracted it years ago, or they themselves could have been carrying it from a previous partner even without knowing it.

You can get an STI from a toilet seat
STIs like warm, moist environments so they wouldn't be able to survive long on a cold toilet seat. Thank goodness!

You can't get an STI from oral sex
STIs are passed through the exchange of bodily fluids (blood, semen, vaginal fluid, eye fluid, breast milk) and skin-to-skin genital contact. Any sexual contact can transmit an STI, including oral and anal sex. The good news is that holding hands, exploring bodies above the waist, kissing, hugging, and sharing food and drinks don't transmit STIs. Teens need to know that.

Not many teens get STIs
Again, STIs don't discriminate. They don't care how old you are. Teens are more likely to get STIs than adults because they generally have higher numbers of sexual partners. In fact, heterosexual girls between the ages of 15 and 24 have the highest rates. This is significant given that some STIs can lead to fertility problems later in life.

Once you get an STI you won't get it again
STIs aren't like chicken pox. Let your teen know that if they test positive, their partner should be treated as well. Otherwise they can just pass the STI back and forth to one another. Plus, a person can be exposed to a certain STI once and then again years later by new partner.

I'd know if I had an STI
If there are any symptoms of an STI, they may include burning when you urinate, a discharge from the penis or vagina, pain during sex, or vaginal odour. But most STIs are asymptomatic, meaning there are no symptoms. You can look healthy and feel healthy, and still have an infection. And you certainly can't tell by looking at someone if they have one. This is why open communication and testing before any sexual contact with a new partner is important.

FUN FACT: Sex workers as a group have some of the lowest STI rates in Canada because they're informed, use condoms consistently, and are tested regularly.

Condoms protect you from all STIs
STIs passed through the exchange of bodily fluids can be prevented by proper, consistent condom use. But unless a person is wearing a full body condom, they don't offer protection against STIs passed through skin-to-skin genital contact (because they don't cover the entire genital area). Other contraceptive methods offer no protection against STIs.

We can get vaccinated against STIs
Only HPV and hepatitis B can be prevented with a vaccination. We don't have vaccines (yet) for any others.

STIs can be cured
Some viral STIs (like HPV in some cases) go away on their own, but not always. You may have them for the rest of your life. Some, like herpes and HIV, can be managed. Bacterial infections can be treated with antibiotics. Some STIs cause infertility or damage to the reproductive system. Others can lead to more serious illnesses, such as cancer. Some, like AIDS, are life-threatening because we don't have a cure.

Getting an STI could kill your sex life forever
Just because you have an STI doesn't mean you can never have sex again. It just requires open communication with your partners and your doctor.

STI tests are painful
Most STI tests are not painful at all. Some require a blood test, but some (for people with a penis) only require a urine sample. Talk about testing and what the procedure looks like. Find out where your teen could go for confidential testing if they don't feel comfortable going to your or their family doctor. Offer to go with them. The best-case scenario, though, would be for them to go with their partner. It's not fair to expect someone else to go for testing if you aren't prepared to go as well. Congratulate your teen for being mature and responsible about this.

TALK SEX TODAY

■ COOL KIDS USE CONTRACEPTION

I know you know this, but I can't help but stress how important it is that we talk to both our daughters and *our sons* about contraception. And, as I mentioned earlier, even if your teen is questioning their sexual attraction, this information is still relevant. Even if your teen has already identified as gay, they may still have vaginal sex at some point. And if they don't, well, at least they can share their knowledge with their friends!

I think most teens today are generally aware of the profound (negative) impact a pregnancy would have on their life at this stage of the game, and I don't think parents need to belabour the point. Yes, there are some teens who get pregnant on purpose, but it's uncommon in the grand scheme of things. More worthwhile would be a conversation or two with your teen to establish that being a parent any time soon isn't in their plans. If you have a son, you'll want to discuss how a pregnancy would affect his life in much the same way as it would his partner's. Once you're on the same page, offer some basic information about how to avoid pregnancy by using contraception.

> *Is there a chance the condom might not work and get her pregnent*

You know I like to share good news, so here's some for you. Based on recent research, SIECAN (The Sex Information and Education Council of Canada) reports that, overall, more and more sexually active young women are using contraception. It's not surprising, then, that the teen pregnancy rate in Canada has been dropping as the rate of contraceptive use among teens has been going up. Yes!

Rather than outline all 20 (yes, there are about 20) contraceptive options and their use and effectiveness, I'd like to focus on the three forms of contraception that are most often used by teens: the external condom (also known as the male condom), oral contraception (also known as OC or birth control pills), and withdrawal (also known as the "pull-out" method). I'd also like to talk about the IUD, a form of contraception that is gaining popularity among young people, and for good reason.

■ EXTERNAL CONDOMS

External condoms are 97% effective at preventing pregnancy and they protect against most STIs if used consistently and as directed. They're also the only contraception that can prevent at least some STIs. They're inexpensive (or are sometimes offered to teens for free) and can be carried around easily.

If you think your teen may be sexually active sometime soon, it's a good idea to have a supply of condoms for them (or their friends). Just put them in the bathroom drawer and let them know they can take them no questions asked. And no, you aren't condoning your teen having sex if you provide condoms, because you are doing it in the context of an ongoing conversation about smart sexual decision-making. Right?

Here are ten things that would be great for your teen to know about external condoms.
1. **Use as directed and practice on yourself** or on your partner before you try it for real. The penis has to be erect when you put it on as well as when you take it off. Make sure there is no air trapped in the tip of the condom once it's on, and leave a half-inch space for semen to be collected.
2. **Optional: Put a drop of water-based lubricant** inside the tip of the condom for increased sensitivity.
3. **Check the expiry date on the package.** If a condom is expired or feels brittle, don't use it. Don't keep condoms in your back pocket because your body heat can break down the latex they're usually made of.
4. **There are novelty (joke) condoms**, and there are condoms that are intended to prevent pregnancy and the spread of STIs. If a con-

dom has Bart Simpson on it and plays "Oh Canada!" or "The Star Spangled Banner" when you unroll it, don't rely on it for anything other than a good laugh.

5. **Always get condoms from a reputable store or clinic**, not from an airport bathroom dispenser. Buy a brand you've heard of.

6. **Condoms are more likely to work if they're lubricated** with a spermicide. If you're using a lubricant separately, make sure it is water-based (oil breaks down latex).

7. **If you or your partner is allergic** to latex, you can buy condoms made of polyurethane or natural materials.

8. **Have the condom talk with your partner** before anything happens. If you get the business out of the way well ahead of time, then you can look forward to the fun!

9. **Don't use two external** – or one external and one internal (female) – condoms at once. Friction can pull them both off.

10. **Unlike other forms of contraception**, condoms can prevent the spread of STIs passed through the exchange of bodily fluids (HIV, hepatitis B and C, gonorrhea, chlamydia). Because they don't cover the entire genital area, though, they offer no protection from STIs that are passed via skin-to-skin-genital contact (HPV, herpes, syphilis). So even if another form of contraception is being used, condoms are a must until you are in a monogamous relationship, your partner is trustworthy, and both of you have tested negative for STIs.

In a perfect world, parents would have the chance to talk to their teen about negotiating condom use with their partner. Like much sexual decision-making, the key is to plan ahead. I joke with teens that they should have the condom talk with their partner not while intertwined on the couch in the heat of the moment, but at Starbucks with a table in between them long before sex is on the menu. Now that's hot.

Suggest to your teen that they keep the conversation with their partner as light-hearted as possible, and that they shouldn't be afraid to admit that they feel awkward, if they do. The message from your teen should be that they want to make sure both they and their partner are safe from STIs and possible pregnancy (if that's relevant). Without the concern of pregnancy or STIs on their minds, sex is going to be a lot more fun for both of them.

Some teens (and adults) will still make the argument that sex doesn't feel as good with a condom, but the latex used these days is so thin it's really not an issue. Plus, some lubricant placed in the tip of the condom can do the trick. If your teen's partner refuses to wear a condom, then your teen needs to think about whether that person is responsible enough to be in a sexual relationship. At the very least, an internal condom can be used.

Of course, teens don't always have sex for the first time in the context of a relationship. They hook up, and the spontaneity of these unions doesn't allow for respectful conversations at Starbucks. This is why your teen should always carry condoms with them if any kind of sex (including oral sex) is even a remote possibility. In that scenario, a simple, "Here, let's use this" will have to do. Whatever the situation, the message needs to be clear that there's no other option.

▄ OC OR "ORAL CONTRACEPTIVE" PILL

The oral contraceptive pill is suitable for people of all ages, can be used long-term, and is 99.9% effective, if used exactly as directed. This makes it the most reliable contraception available. There are two kinds of oral contraceptives: the combined oral contraceptive (COC), and the progestin-only oral contraceptive (POP). While both types have advantages, teens are more likely to be prescribed COC. For this reason, I will focus on COC, but much of the information I'm giving you applies to both kinds.

COC contains estrogen and progestin and prevents pregnancy in three ways: it stops ovulation, it thickens the cervical mucus making it more difficult for sperm to reach an egg, and it changes the lining of the uterus to make implantation of a fertilized egg more difficult.

FUN FACT:
According to www.sexualityandu.ca, the oral contraceptive pill (OC) is one of the world's most prescribed medications, with 100 million women relying on it today.

Here are ten things that would be great for your teen to know about OC.

1. **It's very effective.** Not having to worrying about an unplanned pregnancy during sex makes it way more enjoyable.

2. **It's fully reversible.** In other words, there aren't any lasting effects on fertility. As soon as you stop taking the pills, you can get pregnant.

3. **It can interact with other medications**, decreasing its effectiveness. Conveniently, the most common medications to be aware of start with the letter "A": anti-inflammatories (ibuprofen), antibiotics, anti-convulsants (seizure medication), and anti-fungals. The herbal supplement St. John's Wort can also interact with OC. Prolonged use of these drugs requires a backup method of contraception.

4. **It doesn't offer *any* protection from STIs**, so condom use is a must in most cases.

5. **Pills need to be taken at the same time every day** to maximize effectiveness. Teens might want to set a reminder on their phone until they're in the habit.

6. **Certain brands can reduce acne.** In fact, many teens take OC solely for this reason.

7. **It regulates periods** and reduces period cramps and other premenstrual annoyances.

8. **Side effects can include irregular bleeding or spotting** (light bleeding between periods, generally nothing to worry about), headaches, breast tenderness, nausea, or emotional ups and downs. These usually stabilize in one to three months. Weight gain is rarely an issue given the minimal amounts of hormones in OC compared to when we were in high school, although myths about that are alive and well.

9. **It reduces the risk** of endometrial, uterine, and ovarian cancers, as well as of non-cancerous breast tumours, ovarian cysts, and osteoporosis. It may increase the risk of certain cancers and blood clots (especially for women who have a personal or family history).

10. **It's legal to use in Canada at any age.** If your teen's family doctor is hesitant to prescribe it, go to a youth or sexual health clinic in your community. The cost is sometimes a bit less at these places, too.

For many teens, OC is a great birth control option. Choosing a method is a personal decision, though, and what may work really well for one teen may not work for another. Is your teen mindful enough to remember to take a pill at the same time every day? Are they often on antibiotics or other medications that could decrease the effectiveness of OC? Family health history may also play a role in the decision. If breast cancer runs in your family, for example, POP (progestin-only) may be a better option than COC, as estrogen may be an issue.

■ WITHDRAWAL, OR "THE PULL-OUT" METHOD

I know it's hard to believe, but some teens rely on withdrawal as a form of contraception. As its name indicates, this involves withdrawing the penis from the vagina before ejaculation. But even if a person has the self-control to pull out before orgasm, pre-ejaculate (pre-cum) contains sperm and can cause pregnancy. The website www.sexuality.ca reports a failure rate of 19% in typical users. That means one in five couples who rely on the "pull-out" method will experience a pregnancy – pretty high stakes, especially for teens. Withdrawal also offers no protection from STIs. Although I guess it's better than nothing, the bottom line is that withdrawal isn't an effective method of contraception.

■ IUDs

Since the 1970s when they were pulled from the market because of complication rates, IUDs (intrauterine devices) have gotten a bad rap. Fears have subsided in recent years, though, and IUDs are now considered to be one of the safest, most effective forms of contraception. In fact, a recent study by the American College of Obstetricians and Gynecologists (ACOG) found that of about 90,000 IUD users between the ages of 15 and 44 – less than 1% – had any complications. Today, the organization recommends IUDs for teens and insists that they're a very safe form of contraception for young people.

An IUD is a small T-shaped device that's inserted inside the uterus by a doctor or health care professional qualified to do so. There are two types of IUDs: the Copper IUD and the hormonal intrauterine system (IUS), also known by the brand names Mirena and Jaydess. Made of copper and plastic, the Copper IUD works by preventing sperm from fertilizing an egg, and by preventing implantation of a fertilized egg in the uterine wall. Copper is used because it's a spermicide (it kills sperm). The IUS is made of plastic only, but contains a small amount of the hormone progesterone (not estrogen). It works by releasing progesterone to thin the uterine lining, thickening cervical mucus to make it more difficult for a sperm to fertilize an egg, and stopping ovulation. Much like oral contraception, IUDs prevent conception, so they're not a form of abortion. They're 99% effective in preventing pregnancy, but they don't offer any protection from STIs.

The decision to use a non-hormonal Copper IUD or a hormonal IUS depends on several factors and should be discussed with a doctor. For example, the Copper IUD may be more suitable for women who are breastfeeding or who have had problems with hormonal methods in the past. The IUS may be a better option for women who have heavy periods and bad cramps. In fact, 20% to 30% of women using the IUS will stop having periods altogether (this side effect isn't harmful). Other possible side effects of IUDs include spotting, perforation of the uterus, or expulsion (it falls out).

I encourage parents to talk to their teen about IUDs as a viable contraceptive option. To get an IUD, a doctor needs to provide a prescription and it's usually purchased by the patient at a pharmacy. It's then brought to the doctor or health care professional qualified to insert it. Insertion can be uncomfortable, but it's quick, and cramps that may follow usually only last a few hours.

Seven good reasons teens may choose an IUD:
1. **It provides five years** of effective pregnancy prevention.
2. **They don't have to worry** about taking a pill at the same time every day.
3. **Although the upfront cost is greater** than other forms of contraception, it is cost-effective over the long term.
4. **It's safe with minimal complications** and some positive side effects, such as lighter bleeding, fewer cramps, and less frequent or no periods.
5. **It doesn't require** regular follow-up with a doctor.
6. **It's more private** than OC; no one will know they have one unless they tell them.
7. **Fertility is restored** as soon as the IUD is removed by a doctor or medical practitioner.

Of course, there are other contraceptive methods available to people of all ages, such as the internal condom, the vaginal ring, and the contraceptive patch. I encourage you to explore these options as well, even though they're not as commonly used by teens as the ones I discuss above.

If your teen is in a heterosexual relationship and sex is imminent, it's not a bad idea to prepare ahead and discuss contraception with your family doctor or a health care professional at a sexual health clinic. You may even want to support your teen in using contraception ahead of time so that they're prepared when the time comes. And you can get emergency contraception (EC) from the pharmacy to have on hand should the need arise. Again, this doesn't mean that you're encouraging your teen to have sex; it's about teaching them to think ahead and take care of their reproductive health.

■ PREGNANCY OPTIONS

Most parents would probably agree that learning that their teen, or their teen's partner, is facing an unplanned pregnancy is upsetting, stressful, and overwhelming, to say the least. This is where years of open, non-judgmental communication with your teen can pay off, and so that hopefully they'll feel comfortable sharing this information with you.

As tough as might be, try to hide your shock and disappointment. Thank them for coming to you, and let them know that you're there to support them in any way you can. This isn't the time for "I told you so," or claims that they have ruined their life. They're going to be making some pretty major decisions in the coming weeks and will need your guidance and rational thinking. Not to mention your unconditional love.

If the pregnancy is only suspected and sex without contraception (or with failed contraception) took place five or less days before, talk to your teen and their partner about getting EC as soon as possible. If it's been longer than five days, confirm the pregnancy with an at-home pregnancy test. If the result is positive, don't rush into presenting options right away. You both may need to sleep on it. Take time to process this new information.

Talk with your teen and their partner about what it would be like to be a young parent. How would it affect their relationship? How would it affect their education? How would their priorities need to shift? Their future goals? Their social life? Talk about adoption and the different types of adoption. While an open adoption would allow them to get updates and photos of the child, a closed adoption wouldn't. Assure your teen that they would be allowed to choose the adoptive family.

Talk about abortion too. In Canada, we've come a long way from the dangerous "back alley" and self-administered procedures that too often led to serious injury and even death. Canadian women today have the right to terminate a pregnancy as part of their reproductive choice. For years now, surgical (therapeutic) abortion has been safe and legal at all ages in Canada. But although it's generally available in hospitals and specialized clinics across the country, access is dangerously limited in smaller, remote communities. More recently, RU-486, which is used for medical abortion (abortion induced by medication rather than by surgery) was approved by Health Canada for use up to 49 days into the pregnancy. Both of these abortion options are safe and effective with no lasting effects on fertility.

As a parent, you'll probably know pretty quickly what you'd like your teen to do. But remember that it's not your decision to make. It's your teen's and their partner's decision. Your job is to provide objective information about options in a supportive environment. Give your teen space to express their feelings as often as possible, so that they feel heard and can take ownership of their decision.

■ KEEPING THEIR BODY HEALTHY: SEXUAL HEALTH EXAMS

Even though we may consider ourselves to be mature adults, going to the doctor can be pretty intimidating, especially if we're going for a sexual health exam. If it's daunting for us as adults, we can imagine what it must feel like for a teen! How can we help them cope?

First, we can make sure our teen has a doctor they feel comfortable with. Don't take it personally, but they may not want go to the same doctor as you. Your daughter may want a female doctor, but maybe not. Let them make that decision. Promise them confidentiality and be sure to tell the doctor about your agreement. Second, walk the talk. Go for your own regular checkups, or whenever necessary. I'm not saying you have to excitedly count down the sleeps until your next Pap smear or testicular exam, but don't complain about it (out loud at least). Finally, we can nix fear of the unknown by telling them what to expect.

I'm going to outline sexual health exams step by step in the next few pages, because I hope this will help you describe the experience to your teen. I do this with the understanding that a person's sex assigned at birth may not be consistent with their gender identity. Also, sexual health exams may vary according to a person's unique reproductive system and genital characteristics.

▪ PEOPLE ASSIGNED MALE AT BIRTH

In my experience, most young males are reluctant to visit a doctor. They tell me that they're scared it will be painful, that they don't know what to expect, and that it will be awkward and embarrassing. Some doctors aren't especially proficient at calming these fears and often rush through the exam in order to lessen the agony. Of course, guys occasionally share the agony with their buddies and then rumours, stories, guilt, and shame are passed along, person-to-person, generation-to-generation.

Here's how Meg and I would explain a routine sexual health exam to a teen assigned male at birth.

First, the doctor should take a medical history. That means you just talk. A good doctor will probably ask you the following questions: Are you healthy? Do you have any general health problems or challenges? Are you sexually active (meaning have you had any kind of sex before, and are you in any sexual relationships right now)? How often do you have sex? Do you have sex with one, or more than one partner? What kind of sex do you have, and, if relevant, what kind of contraception do you and your partner(s) use? How do you feel about the sexual experiences you've had? Do you have any pain/questions/concerns at the moment?

Doctors shouldn't assume that you're heterosexual or exclusively gay. They should also listen to your answers attentively. Be honest so that the doctor can best meet your needs, but if you feel uncomfortable or judged, then maybe this isn't the right doctor for you.

Next, the doctor will need to examine your genitals, so you have to take your pants off. You should be given a gown or an examining drape to cover yourself. The doctor may cup your scrotum with their hand, feel your testicles, and ask you to cough. They do this to check the health of your testicles. Do they move when you cough? Are they smooth? Are there any lumps, bruises, warts, sores, or swelling? And the doctor should teach you how to do a testicular self-exam too. (You get bonus points if you already do this at least once a month.)

In case you're not having enough fun yet, the doctor will look at your penis for any similar problems, and to see if there is any abnormal discharge (moisture coming out of the urethra).

It's really important that you're honest with your doctor about the sexual activities you've engaged in so that they can give you the best care possible. If you have had anal sex, for example, they may also swab your anus.

Remember that STIs can be spread by skin-to-skin genital contact and the exchange of body fluids. That includes needle sharing and getting tattoos or piercings with unclean instruments. Your doctor may also do an abdominal exam, checking your liver and spleen in particular for signs of infection. Blood tests may be ordered.

A thorough sexual health checkup takes about 15 minutes. If you've never had sex (of any kind) and are healthy in all other respects, it would be a good idea to start going for this exam when you're 18 or 19 years old. If all is good, you may not need to go again until you enter a sexual relationship. Then you'll need to go for an exam with each new sexual partner, or if you find out that your relationship isn't exclusive.

And remember: if you feel judged, uncomfortable, or that your doctor isn't taking your concerns seriously, trust your gut and find a new one.

▌ PEOPLE ASSIGNED FEMALE AT BIRTH

A thorough gynecological exam involves both a pelvic exam to check the ovaries and uterus, as well as a Pap smear. A Pap smear is when the doctor takes a sample of cells from the cervix (the opening to the uterus) to check for abnormal cells that might indicate cervical cancer. Although they vary slightly from province to province, current Canadian recommendations for gynecological exams generally state that they should start at age 21, or within three years of first sexual contact. Pap smears should be done annually until there are three consecutive years of negative results. At that point, they should be done every two years until the age of 70.

Here's how I would describe a routine sexual health exam to a teen assigned female at birth.

First, the doctor should take a medical history. That means you just talk. The doctor will probably ask you the same questions they ask everyone: Are you healthy? Do you have any general health problems or challenges? Are you sexually active (meaning have you had any kind of sex before, and are you in any sexual relationships right now)? How often do you have sex? Do you have sex with one, or more than one partner? What kind of sex do you have and, if relevant, what contraception do you and your partner(s) use? How do you feel about the sexual experiences you have had? Do you have any pain/questions/concerns at the moment?

Doctors should not assume that you are heterosexual or exclusively gay. They should also listen to your answers attentively. Be honest so that the doctor can best meet your needs, but if you feel uncomfortable or judged, then maybe this isn't the right doctor for you.

Next, the doctor will probably leave you so you can get undressed for the exam. When they come back into the room, you'll be asked to lie on your back on the examining table and to put your heels up, next to your buttocks. Often doctors ask patients to put their feet up in stirrups for the exam, but they're not mandatory. If you'd rather keep your feet on the table, you can always ask the doctor to do the exam without stirrups. It's your decision.

Here's where the real fun begins. The doctor will use a plastic or metal instrument called a speculum so that they can see inside your vagina. If it's a metal speculum, you can ask the doctor to run it under warm water before inserting it. Trust me, it's way more comfortable that way! Once the doctor has inserted the speculum, they can expand it a bit to look at your vagina. It should look pink, moist, and healthy, just like the inside of your cheek – only more wrinkled. Then the doctor will take a wooden stick (a bit like a tongue depressor) and scrape a few cells off your cervix, the entrance to the uterus. Those cells get wiped onto a glass slide and are sent to a cytology lab where they're tested for cancer or pre-cancerous cells. This procedure is called a Pap smear, and it only takes a minute. It doesn't test for STIs.

If you've ever had digital, anal, oral, or vaginal sex it's a good idea to get checked for STIs every time you have a new sexual partner. It's easy to test for some STIs at the same time as a Pap smear, but don't assume your doctor is doing that. Always request STI screening specifically if you have had any new sexual relationships since your last visit. It's hard to believe, but doctors sometimes make assumptions about STI risk and do testing based on age, relationship status, and sexual attraction.

For example, suspecting her husband was having an affair, someone I know worked up the courage to ask her doctor for STI testing. He replied, "Why would you need to be tested, you've been married for 12 years!" At that point she just shut down and left the office. The reasons for wanting and needing STI testing vary greatly. Maybe the person has just heard that a previous partner has tested positive for an STI. Or maybe *they've* had an affair. You never know, right?

Certain STI tests require a sample of cells from the cervix as well, and this can be done right after the Pap smear while the speculum is still in. The doctor will swab the cervix again with two cotton swabs. The swabs go to a different lab to check for STIs.

After removing the speculum, the doctor will then put on a latex glove and insert two fingers into your vagina; the doctor's other hand goes on your abdomen. This procedure is called the pelvic exam, which means the doctor is checking for abnormalities in the uterus and ovaries. This part of the exam literally takes less than a minute.

Before you go, you may be asked for urine and blood samples as well. Some STIs are tested using blood, and urine can offer information about things like sugar (glucose) and protein in the body. A urine sample is *not* a good indicator of STIs because the urine doesn't come out of the vagina. While you're there, the doctor should also check for

[Handwritten note: What is a pap smear?]

breast lumps and will review the breast self-examination that you should do monthly. There's some controversy about whether breast self-exams are necessary, but I think we should always know what our breasts look and feel like, and we can notice any changes that way.

TIPS FOR TALKING TO TEENS

Keep your eye on the prize: a happy, healthy, sexually-mature adult. With each conversation, your teen is moving in that direction.

Check your baggage. Don't expect your teen to do what you did or didn't do sexually when you were younger. Maybe they will, but maybe they won't. And that may be a good thing!

Don't buy into the parental paranoia that all teens today are sexting during class, giving blow jobs in the bathroom at nutrition break, and having massive orgies on the weekend. Think critically about what you hear, and remember that statistics report averages and can often be misleading. Benchmarks are helpful, but may not characterize your teen.

Don't share information about your personal sexual experiences if you aren't comfortable doing so. We all have different comfort zones, and some topics feel off limits. Simply explain that you'd rather not talk about your own sexual experiences. And promise that you won't ask your teen about their sexual experiences either when they're adults.

(I know, it's hard enough to get your head around them having sex, never mind talking about it!)

No lecturing. Don't say things like, "You're not giving blow jobs in the bathroom like other girls in your school, are you?" or "You know that having sex before you're married can lead to all kinds of problems, right?" Guaranteed fail. Instead, let your teen take the lead. Do more listening than talking, and when you *do* talk, ask lots of questions like, **"How did that make you feel?" "Can you tell me more about that?" "What do you think works best for you?" "Do many people your age feel that way?" "Was there anything to learn from that experience?"**

Along the same lines, don't start the conversation with, "We need to talk." Your teen will immediately assume they're in trouble and will be on the defensive.

Break down important conversations into manageable chunks. (It's not about the two-hour-tell-all.) Grab every chance you can get – in the car, while walking the dog, during commercial breaks....

Avoid eye contact if you need to.

And after that, you're done! I'd be lying if I said that I look forward to my regular Pap smear and pelvic exam. They aren't painful, but I would describe them as uncomfortable. I find that it helps to stay as relaxed as possible and to remember that what I am doing could save

(I can't believe I just wrote that.) You might be able to keep your teen engaged for longer and delve into tougher topics if they don't have to look you right in the eyes. Side by side – for example, while exploring an educational website for teens, or power walking – may be more comfortable and productive. I've had the best conversations with my stepdaughters after school in the kitchen while I'm prepping dinner and they're making a snack. Focusing on something else seems to make conversation easier. Plus nothing beats multitasking.

Don't rule out text and email as valid ways to share information and discuss issues with your teen. (I can't believe I wrote that one either.) Of course, nothing replaces face-to-face conversations, but texting a link to an article, for example, could lead to some interesting back-and-forth.

Use language you feel comfortable with, language that's "you." If you wouldn't otherwise use words or phrases like "be intimate," "heavy petting," "courting," and "give your virginity," don't use them with your teen. You'll lose them. You'll also lose your teen if you try to be *too* cool by using teen slang. Leave the "shipping" and "slaying" for them and their friends.

Be honest. If you don't know the meaning of a slang word your teen asks about, go to **www.urbandictionary.com** and report back. No one expects you to know everything about sex, just have good resources handy.

If your teen brings something up (for example, Sarah and I are thinking about having sex) just as you're about to get on a conference call, thank them for sharing that and tell them you'd love to talk more about it, and *will*, when you get off the call. Even if you're not getting on a conference call, be honest if you need a bit of time to respond. Gather your thoughts, call your sister for moral support, and revisit the comment later when you're feeling less flustered. If you're nervous, flustered, or seem totally uncomfortable when your teen asks a question, they'll pick up on it and won't come to you with their next question because it's awkward. They can smell your fear.

Continued over ...

my life. For real. As an adult, I don't feel the slightest bit anxious about the visit, but it's totally normal if you do, especially before your first few exams. Bring a friend (or your mom or your sister) or ask a nurse hold your hand during the exam. Seriously! And don't forget to congratulate yourself after for being so mature, and responsible, and brave. You're taking great care of your body.

The whole examination usually takes 15 to 30 minutes, but you can always ask for more time. Don't be afraid or too embarrassed to ask questions or to ask for explanations. You're entitled to choices and to a full understanding of why you may be asked certain questions, and why specific procedures have to be done. Besides, doctors usually like it when teens care and know enough to ask them questions. If you have lots and lots and lots of questions, the doctor may book another appointment.

At the same time, don't miss opportunities to talk with your teen because the timing isn't perfect. Pick up on their cues and stay on your toes. If they loiter in the kitchen while you unpack groceries, chances are they need money or a ride. But chances are also good they want to talk to you about something important.

Be breezy (think Monica from *Friends*). Despite your understandable inner freak-out, never let your teen see it. If you want them to open up to you, have a mature conversation with you, or actually absorb the information you're trying to give them, you need to pull yourself together and act like there's nothing you'd rather be talking about. Also, sometimes teens take great pleasure from watching us squirm. Let's not give them that satisfaction. You got this.

Get back on that horse. If one conversation goes down like a lead balloon, get yourself up, brush yourself off, and ask yourself what will work better next time. Was it bad timing? Was it too lecture-like? Did you talk too much? Were they just not in the mood? Were you just not in the mood? Don't take rejection personally. It's not you, it's the topic. Plus you're dealing with a hormonal teen.

Make sure your alone time together isn't *always* attached to a discussion of this agenda. Otherwise they'll start to dread hanging out with you.

■ ADOLESCENT CHECKLIST (GRADES 8-12)

Your adolescent child needs to know everything the previous age groups have learned. They should also know

- about sexual consent and how to express their boundaries assertively
- how to cope with a breakup
- the proper use of condoms, oral contraception, and IUDs
- about STIs
- about the availability of and have access to community sexual health resources
- pregnancy options
- what to expect during a sexual health examination

They should also have

- a deeper understanding of healthy versus unhealthy relationships
- relationship and sexual decision-making skills, as well as effective communication skills
- safety agreements for going to parties

And they should understand

- the pressure placed on teens to be sexually active
- their personal sexuality-related values and boundaries
- the impact of our hypersexualized society

RESOURCES

FOR PARENTS

WEBSITES
- www.optbc.org
- www.sexualityandu.ca
- www.scarleteen.com

BOOKS
- *Breaking the Hush Factor: Ten Rules for Talking with Teenagers about Sex*, by Dr. Karen Rayne See also www.breakingthehushfactor.com
- *Masterminds and Wingmen: Helping Our Boys Cope with Schoolyard Power, Locker-Room Tests, Girlfriends, and the New Rules of Boy World*, by Rosalind Wiseman.
- *Queen Bees and Wannabes: Helping Your Daughter Survive Cliques, Gossip, Boyfriends, and the New Realities of Girl World*, by Rosalind Wiseman.
- *Talking to Your Kids about Sex: Turning "The Talk" into a Conversation for Life*, by Dr. Laura Berman.

FOR TEENS

WEBSITES AND YOUTUBE CLIPS
- www.optbc.org
- www.sexualityandu.ca
- www.scarleteen.com
- www.womancareglobal.org ("If You Don't Tell Them, Then Who Will?" Actor Jessica Biel teaches sex education)
- www.youtube.com/user/lacigreen (a frank video series about sexuality with young adult sex educator Laci Green)

- www.blush.vch.ca (a website created by Vancouver Coastal Health based on the workshops they offer in high schools addressing sexuality, media literacy, healthy relationships and gender stereotypes)
- www.gurl.com
- www.makelovenotporn.com (a website that compares pornography with "real" sex)
- www.sexetc.org
- www.kidshelpphone.ca

BOOKS

- *Changing Bodies, Changing Lives: A Book for Teens on Sex and Relationships*, by Ruth Bell.
- *Deal With It! A Whole New Approach to Your Body, Brain, and Life as a Gurl*, by E. Drill, H. McDonald, and R. Odes (the creators of gurl.com).
- *S.E.X.: The All-You-Need-To-Know Progressive Sexuality Guide to Get You through High School and College*, by Heather Corinna.
- *The Guy Book: A User's Manual*, by Mavis Jukes.
- *The New Teenage Body Book*, by Kathy McCoy and Dr. Charles Wibbelsman

12. Straight Answers to Sticky Questions

12. Straight Answers to Sticky Questions

At the end of my evening sessions, parents often approach me privately to ask questions they "wouldn't dare" ask in front of the group. Most of these have to do with questions their children have asked, but they have no idea how to answer. And who can blame them?

Our kids throw us some real doozies from time to time! This chapter is meant to help you get your head around some of the tougher questions your kids might ask, *before* they ask them. Before we dive in, though, here are a few tips to keep in your back pocket.

When your child asks you a tough question, don't freak out. Or at least, try not to. Remind yourself that they're giving you a huge compliment. Your child trusts you as a credible and approachable source of sexual health information. Take a deep breath and keep your voice neutral. The goal is to stay as calm as a cucumber without getting angry or sounding shocked.

If you can't think of an answer right away (which is both understandable and completely acceptable), tell your child, **"I'm glad you asked me that question and you deserve a scientific answer. But let me think about how best to answer you and we'll talk about it before bed (or when our guests leave, or when we walk the dog later, or when your little sister goes to bed)."** Be honest about your discomfort, but don't let it get in the way of taking advantage of this great opportunity to give information.

When you answer the question, you might want to start by asking your child where they heard that word or why they are wondering about the question. This can give you some useful context. Then, give some basic scientific information and watch for their reaction. Are they looking at you expectantly, needing more information? Or are they on to their next question about something totally different? If so, enough said.

DO YOU AND MOM (DAD) STILL HAVE SEX?

Personally, I think we need to do a better job of celebrating sexual activity in any healthy, adult, consenting relationship. There really is no reason that parents should hide the fact that they have sex. Kids need to know that parents who love each other usually have sex too.

The fact that their parents have sex isn't really a surprise to most children. I meet so many kids who have a pretty good idea what happens when they go to bed, or on Saturday mornings (isn't that what iPads and cartoons are for?). But they often feel anxiety around their parents having sex. Parents who have had the misfortune of a little one walking in on them tell me that their child's main concern is that someone is getting hurt. We can't blame them; it would be pretty scary to see one parent on top of the other…or worse!

When students disclose to me that their parents have sex, I'm always careful to tell them how lucky they are to have parents who love each other. Any anxiety or sense of being grossed-out they may have displayed in the disclosure is quickly replaced with relief. Of course, I also say, **"Some kids have parents who aren't in a relationship so they may not be having sex right now. But most parents hope that one day they'll have someone else have to sex with, because they think that having sex is a great thing."** That comforts children with single parents who may or may not be in a new relationship.

Parents have different comfort levels in terms of how much of their sex life they're willing to share with their kids, and there's no right or wrong way to answer personal questions. Just make sure you don't lie. You may feel okay talking about the value of sex in your relationship.

And when your child asks if they can watch you and your partner do it, an appropriate answer is, "No, it's private." Other parents may explain to their child that their curiosity is normal, but that having sex is private so they don't want to talk about their personal experiences. The deal, of course, is that they need to promise their child they won't ask details about *their* sex life when they are adults either!

Remember that young children are usually quite blasé about the whole sex thing, like my friend's six-year-old son. After visiting his Grade 1 class, a friend called to tell me about their conversation on the way home from school. Soon after getting in the car, her son shared

> Is there an age limit to have sex? (can you be too old?)

that I had taught them how babies are usually made through sex. He then asked her, "So do you and Dad still do that?" My friend took a deep breath and simply said, "Yes," to which he replied, "Okay, that's fine, but just don't do it on my bed!"

DID YOU HAVE SEX BEFORE YOU WERE MARRIED? HOW MANY PEOPLE HAVE YOU HAD SEX WITH?

Again, the answer to these personal questions really depends on a parent's comfort level and sense of privacy. But being honest is key. A parent may say, **"Yes, I did have sex before I was married (or "I've had many sexual partners"), but I didn't have the same information young people today have about the responsibilities that come with it. You'll make smarter decisions then we did growing up because you're better informed."** Keep in mind that if your teen asks this question, it's possible that what they're really asking is, "Is it okay to have sex right now?" This is when communicating your family values and beliefs about sex comes in. Children and teens need to know where parents stand so it can guide their behaviour. And believe it or not, they *like* having these boundaries.

CAN PEOPLE IN A WHEELCHAIR HAVE SEX?

Start by acknowledging to your child that their curiosity is normal. But you can't tell by looking at a person in a wheelchair (or on crutches, or walking with an obvious physical disability) if they can have sex. Some people who are severely disabled have full sexual function and are capable (with assistance) of having sex and reproducing. Some people who are disabled cannot. Especially with little ones, we should stress that, although we're very pleased they're curious enough to ask us this question, it wouldn't be polite to ask a person who's disabled about their sexual functioning. Gotta teach good manners and boundaries!

WHAT ABOUT NUDITY AT HOME?

This isn't a question kids usually ask, but it's a question I get from parents *all the time*. Specifically, parents want to know how much nudity in the home is "normal," when should parents and children (or siblings) stop bathing together, and is there an age cut-off? The general wisdom these days is that whoever says "No" rules. Many parents and children feel just fine bathing or showering together and most siblings love to bath together, especially in the preschool and early primary years. Enjoy it while it lasts, because it won't last forever! Sometimes it's the parent who begins to feel uncomfortable or simply crowded out as the children grow bigger. That's when the parent can say, **"I'd like to have my bath or shower alone from now on. I need my privacy."** This is amazing role modelling by the parent. It gives their child permission to say the same thing when it becomes important for them to have their privacy.

The situation would be the same for siblings who've enjoyed sharing a bath. When one says, "I don't want to do this anymore," or "I want to bath by myself tonight," that child rules. It's really important that the parent support the child and respect their developing boundaries. Sometimes a younger child will become shy before an older one does, or will want privacy one day, but not another day. They're not just testing their parents; they're testing themselves and their own boundaries. Parents need to just roll with it as much as possible.

WHAT'S A BLOW JOB, A BJ, A 69? WHAT IS ORAL SEX, ANAL SEX, KINKY SEX, FINGER-BANGING?

I know, I know. Take a minute to catch your breath. These questions can be particularly shocking to parents who aren't aware that exposure to these topics happens at increasingly younger ages. The reality is that kids are exposed to all things sexual much sooner than we'd like to think. So how do we tackle these gems?

First, if the question is asked at the dinner table with your child using a guest as a shield, don't be afraid to use the old, "That's a good question; we'll talk before bed" trick. Be prepared, though, that if you have normal friends and relatives they'll all want to stay for bedtime to hear your answer! And don't pay too much attention to a sexually immature friend who suggests that you wash your child's mouth out with soap.

Second, as always, remember that questions are a compliment. Your child trusts you to give an honest answer. Honour the question and the courage it took to ask.

Third, be grateful for the time you've got now to think about what you want to say.

Then, bring on the science and health information. Replace their slang with scientific terms. For example, if they've asked, "What's a blow job?" you could say, **"It's a slang term for oral sex. Have you heard of oral sex before? Oral sex is when someone's mouth is placed on someone's genitals. Specifically, a blow job (also known as a BJ) is when someone's mouth is placed on someone's penis. Sixty-nine (69) refers to a sexual position that partners can use when they perform oral sex on each other."** Your child's response will probably be to cover their ears and scream, "Eww, gross! Why would anyone want to do that?!" Simply respond with, **"You never have to have oral sex if you don't want to. It's normal for kids your age to think it's gross because it's not appropriate for kids to do."**

Here's what you could say about anal sex. **"Anal sex is when some-**

one's penis is placed in someone's anus. Sometimes men who have sex with men do that, and sometimes men do that while having sex with women. In a healthy relationship, both partners consent to any kind of sex they're having, and whoever says 'No' rules."

In recent months, more and more students are asking me about "kinky sex." I explain that the word "kinky" generally refers to something that's out of the ordinary or unusual, so kinky sex refers to ways of having sex that are maybe not as common in the general population. Kinky sex may involve sex toys, fantasy, and role-playing.

"Finger-banging (or fingering) is a slang word for digital sex, which involves someone's finger(s) either stimulating the clitoris or being placed in someone's vagina or anus." Now here comes more science and health information. First, if fingers are inserted into the anus, they shouldn't later be inserted into the vagina because this can give a person an infection. Second, fingering typically doesn't cause pregnancy. In order to make a baby during sex, sperm needs to join an egg, usually through the vagina. You can also point out that if sperm are swallowed or placed in the anus, they will come out as stool. If you happen to be dealing with a primary-aged child, you're back to their favourite subject and they'll be rolling on the floor in hysterical laughter.

If one or both partners have an STI, the bacteria or virus can be transferred from the genitals or fingers, anus or mouth, to the other person. Most bacteria and viruses will grow wherever there is a mucous membrane. So it's possible to have STIs growing in the throat, mouth, eyes, anus, and any part of the genitals. Help your child understand the importance of regular STI testing and being honest with their partner(s) and their doctor about which kinds of sex they've had.

I ask teens to ask themselves, "Do I feel comfortable going to the doctor for testing? Can I be honest with my doctor about my sexual activities?" And most important, "Could I tell my partner if I had an infection?" If their answer is an agonized, "Um no, I'd rather die," then I suggest that they rethink whether they're ready for a sexual relationship. Come to think of it, more adults should be asking themselves these questions too!

To end the conversation on a positive note, remind your child that sex between two consenting adults in a healthy relationship is a great thing. *Consenting* is the key word. Partners should decide *together* what kinds of sex they would like to have, if any at all.

WHAT ARE SEX TOYS?

After you pick your jaw up off the floor, ask your child where they heard this term or why they'd like to know. Once you've got some context, explain that, **"a sex toy is an object or device used for sexual stimulation or to enhance sexual pleasure and fun. People can enjoy using sex toys alone or with a partner."** Specifically (because they are most likely to ask about this), **"a dildo is made of silicone, plastic, or rubber and is usually shaped a bit like an erect penis. If it has a battery in it to make it vibrate, it is called a vibrator."**

Legally, sex toys can only be sold to adults, not to children. And, when they're an adult, they can decide to use them, or not. It's a personal choice. As long as they're clean, sex toys are perfectly healthy and safe to use. *Clean* is the key word, though, because some viruses, especially hepatitis, can survive for long periods of time on sex toys and are capable of infecting or re-infecting the user.

DOES CAITLYN JENNER STILL HAVE TESTICLES?

This question demonstrates how much our children absorb from the media around them – a good reminder that kids are exposed to more than we think, sooner than we think. And what a perfect, teachable moment to talk about people who are transgender! Even with very young children, we can explain that sometimes a person's gender identity isn't consistent with the sex they were assigned at birth. Simply

> *What does 69 mean?*
>
> *Does 96 mean anything?*

put, how someone feels as a boy or a girl on the inside sometimes doesn't match how they look on the outside. For example, a person may feel like a girl, but be perceived by other people as a boy. This is called being transgender. For some people, their gender identity doesn't fit neatly into one of those two choices. They may feel both male and female, or like something entirely different. ("Something entirely different" may include people who identify as "gender fluid," "genderqueer," "non-binary," or "non-conforming" to name a few options, but not all.) These are all examples of how gender is complex and how all of us are unique. The important thing is that we respect and celebrate these differences.

> *What happens if the boy puts his Penis in the wrong hole?*

If they choose, people who are transgender can transition from male to female, or from female to male. This process may or may not involve treatments, medication, and surgery to change the body physically. It's up to the person to decide. As for the whether Caitlin Jenner still has testicles, who knows? It's really none of our business. The decision to alter a person's body is a very personal one. Besides, what matters is that the person themselves feels good about how their body looks underneath their clothes, and that we support the unique challenges that transgender people face.

WHAT'S A HOOKER? WHAT'S A "HO"?

The slang terms "hooker" and "ho" (as well as "prostitute") are disrespectful words for a sex worker. The more general term "sex worker" is preferable, to avoid reinforcing the stigma associated with the other terms above.

A sex worker is someone (of any gender) who exchanges sex for money. Unfair stereotypes portray sex workers as down-and-out types who sell their bodies solely out of desperation to support a drug or alcohol addiction. The common assumption is that they live on the street, come from dysfunctional homes, and are riddled with sexually transmitted infections. It's time we question these stereotypes and tell our children the truth. Yes, some sex workers do what they do because they're desperate or feel that they have no other means of survival. But many *choose* this work.

Rather than comment on the moral value or legality of sex work, a more meaningful approach would include discussion of issues affecting sex workers in our communities. For example, Pace Society (www.pace-society.org), an organization dedicated to giving programs and services to sex workers in Vancouver, British Columbia, educates the public about how sex workers are negatively impacted by sex work criminalization, policing strategies, stigma and discrimination, racism and transphobia.

WHY ARE PEOPLE GAY? HOW DO YOU KNOW IF SOMEONE'S GAY? HOW DO GAY PEOPLE "DO IT"?

It's hard to believe that once upon a time in human history, babies who were born as twins or triplets were killed because they were considered bad luck. Children who were born left-handed (that would be me!) were beaten or killed because it was believed that they were possessed by Satan. And children who had red hair or who retained their blue eyes after birth were abandoned as "devils." Of course, all of the above is superstitious garbage, and we've matured enough to understand that about 10% of any population will be born left-handed, blue-eyed, or as part of a multiple birth.

I don't think it's useful to belabour the question of *why* people are gay. A parent might want to start with, **"No one knows exactly what determines who we are sexually attracted to, just like no one knows why some people are left-handed."** It might be helpful to add that people used to believe it was "caused" by something that happened to a child, such as an absent father, not enough hormones, or abuse. Now we know that homosexuality is not something you can "catch," it's not a lifestyle that someone "chooses," and that a person's romantic and sexual attraction is already in place at birth. There's also some evidence that it's genetic. But regardless of who a person wants to share their sexuality with, *we're all human first.*

I understand and respect that different families have different values and beliefs about homosexuality. But I can't think of one religion that doesn't teach that all people deserve respect. No one has the right to call us names or to discriminate against us because of our romantic or sexual attraction, race, religion, or anything else. The reality, though, is that homophobia (and transphobia) is killing our kids. Suicides among teens and young adults are often related to fears around sexual attraction – fears that are exacerbated by homophobic putdowns, harassment, and jokes. Too many young men are afraid to masturbate or to do testicular self-exams for fear that touching themselves means they're gay. And too many teens are trying to prove that they are straight, by engaging in heterosexual sex and becoming pregnant long before they're ready for those responsibilities.

The truth is, when I explain to five-year-olds that being gay (or homosexual) means to be romantically or sexually attracted to someone of the same sex, they look at me as if to say, "Yah, tell us something we don't know!" In terms of answering the questions of older kids about how gay people have sex, we can simply explain that there are many different kinds of sex (see above) and that they don't all involve a penis and vagina. Regardless of whether people are gay, straight, somewhere in between, or something entirely different, consenting adults in a healthy relationship would decide together which kinds of sex they want to have, if any at all.

When it comes to how you can tell whether someone's gay, the easy answer is, "You can't." We need to get rid of dangerous and inac-

> Why are some people gay and others not?

> How do i know if im gay or not?

curate stereotypes that teach people that gay people look, dress, talk, or act in certain ways. As for how someone would know that they themselves are gay, it's a different experience for everyone. Some know from the day they're born; others take years to explore and truly understand their romantic and sexual attraction. And for many people, their attraction is fluid. It changes over time. Whatever the case, we need to not just accept, but *celebrate* and *nurture* these human differences. When it comes to doing this, our five-year-olds have much to teach us!

> What does mean. to be a virgin? Or how to lose virginity

WHAT DOES IT MEAN TO LOSE YOUR VIRGINITY? HOW CAN YOU TELL IF A PERSON IS A VIRGIN?

Although it does come up from time to time, students are asking me less and less about the concept of virginity, because we seldom use the term these days. This makes me happy, because I think it's outdated and useless for a few reasons.

First, the concept of virginity has been based on misinformation about anatomy. When I first started teaching in the late '90s, a virgin was simply defined as a person who had never had vaginal sex. It was also assumed that first-time vaginal sex would tear the hymen and cause bleeding. If a woman didn't bleed the first time she had vaginal sex, then clearly she wasn't a virgin.

We now know that this isn't true. Some girls are born without a hymen, and some hymens get torn and stretched painlessly and without bleeding long before sexual contact. Stories about woman having their "cherry popped" the first time they have vaginal sex are garbage. That ugliness is much more about ignorance of anatomy than about virginity.

I also have a problem with the concept of virginity because it's too simplistic. That is, it doesn't take into account the different kinds of sex a person may have and makes the assumption that vaginal sex is the be-all and end-all. What if a person has never had vaginal sex but has had oral sex countless times? Are they still a virgin?

I also find the concept of "losing" one's virginity very "sex negative." In a healthy, consenting sexual relationship, there's nothing to *lose* and lots to *gain* – like pleasure, intimacy, fun, stress relief, and physical and emotional connection with another person.

I think it's worth letting our children know that no one, not even a doctor, can say with absolute certainty whether a person has or has not had vaginal sex. Of course, the presence of sperm or semen, STI organisms, or bruising and tearing in or around the vagina may be an indication of vaginal sex. But maybe not. Pregnancy can happen without penetration and isn't an indicator that someone has had vaginal sex. Besides, who cares if a person is a virgin? If a person wants you to know about the kinds of sex they have or haven't had, they'll tell you! End of story.

WHY DO PEOPLE MAKE NOISE WHEN THEY HAVE SEX?

The easy answer to this question is, **"They don't always. Sometimes sex is very quiet and peaceful."** But children often get the impression that sex is noisy because of what they see on TV, in movies, and, unfortunately, in pornography. In these unrealistic portrayals, there's a lot of noise, moans, heavy breathing, sweating, groaning, shouting, even screaming during sex. As a result, it's not unusual for children ask me, "Why does the lady scream when you do it to her?" "Why do people moan?" and sadly, "Why do you have to beat the lady before you do it?"

Please talk to your kids about the difference between entertainment and reality, and about how sex is exaggerated in entertainment to get viewers' attention and money. Unfortunately, some people mimic what they see in media, thinking the Hollywood version of sex is the norm. For sexually mature adults in a healthy, consenting relationship, sex isn't always dramatic; it's not a competition, it's not a marathon, and it doesn't require academy award-winning performances. Amen to that!

WHAT IS AN ORGASM? CAN A WOMAN HAVE A BUNCH IN A ROW?

For most men, an orgasm involves semen (the fluid that carries sperm) being ejaculated from their penis. After ejaculation, their body relaxes and the penis goes back to its usual size. For most women, an orgasm involves contractions of the muscles around the vagina, and sometimes around the uterus and anus. Although women don't ejaculate in the same way that men do, some women experience a kind of ejaculation of vaginal fluid.

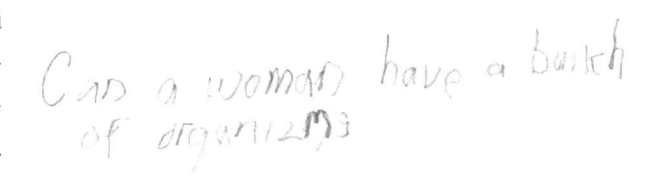

For reproduction purposes, the contraction of the vaginal muscles during orgasm is intended to pull ejaculated sperm up, deeper into the vagina to increase the chances that sperm will reach and fertilize an egg. But because it's not always a man and woman having sex, not to mention reproduction is usually not the goal of sex, the purpose of orgasm is more often for pleasure. It's the part of sexual activity that feels the best. Some people associate it with the tension you feel when you're about to sneeze. An orgasm is a release of that tension, but it feels a million times better.

I think it's really important to explain to older children and teens that sex can be fun and feel good even without an orgasm. Also, more often than not, partners may not have an orgasm at the same time. Typically, men become sexually aroused and reach orgasm faster than women. But it also depends on other factors, such as arousal level, health issues, stress, how a person feels toward their partner, how tired they are, and whether they have consumed alcohol or cigarettes. And one partner may orgasm, but the other may not.

As for a woman having "a bunch" of orgasms in a row, many women can. And many women can't. Coming from a preteen or teen, though, I can't help but think this question stems from watching or at least hearing what happens in pornography. Again, let's remind our kids that sex in entertainment usually doesn't look like that in real life.

HOW EXACTLY DOES THE PENIS GET INTO THE VAGINA?

There are lots of different ways that the penis can enter the vagina. But regardless of how partners may position themselves during sex, they put their bodies very close together, usually with their clothes off, in a private place like a bedroom. When the penis is getting ready to deliver sperm, it gets hard. A hard penis is called an erection, and it enables the penis to enter the vagina quite easily. Sexual arousal can produce moisture in the vagina, which acts as a lubricant and makes it slippery, and that makes it easier for the penis to enter too. Sometimes people may guide the penis into the vagina with their hands, but that's not always necessary.

WHY DO PEOPLE REMOVE THE HAIR ON THEIR GENITALS? SHOULD I DO IT BEFORE I HAVE SEX?

Given that we live in a society where you can walk down the street and see sandwich boards offering "Brazilians" and "manscaping," and that views body hair as repulsive, it's not surprising that kids ask questions about hair removal. When answering, start by explaining the science of pubic hair – that it's protection for the genitals. Much like we have eye lashes to keep the germs out of our eyes, and hair in our nostrils to keep the germs out of our nose, pubic hair acts as a screen for the genitals. So scientifically speaking, there is no health reason to remove *any* of our body hair. In fact, most people in the world don't.

But in Western culture, children see women at the beach and it's not difficult to notice that there's no hair sticking out of their bikini bottoms. Some children are exposed to pornography online and see pretty clearly that no one has pubic hair (or any other body hair for that matter).

Pubic hair is important, but people can choose whether they want to remove or shape it. When it comes to sex, though, removing pubic hair is by no means a prerequisite.

WHAT IS THE G-SPOT?

According to Wikipedia, the G-spot (or Gräfenberg spot) is a sensitive area of the vagina that, when stimulated, may lead to strong sexual arousal, powerful orgasms, and potential ejaculation. It's believed to be located two to three inches inside, on the upper or front vaginal wall. But despite research on the G-spot since the 1940s, its existence has never been proven, nor has the source of vaginal ejaculation. We know from subjective reports, though, that some people absolutely believe it's the secret to mind-blowing sexual pleasure. As a result, many couples spend a good chunk of their intimate time on a quest to find it.

When it comes to talking to our kids about the G-spot, I think more meaningful than debating its existence or prevailing theories on how to find it would be a conversation about sexual pleasure in general. Whether the G-spot is real or not doesn't really matter. There are lots of ways that people with vaginas can feel pleasure – feeling abnormal or inadequate because you can't find the supposed sweet spot just gets in the way of enjoying them!

13. Teaching Sexual Health to Children and Teens with Special Needs

13. Teaching Sexual Health to Children and Teens with Special Needs

I couldn't write a book about sexual health for kids without including this important chapter. I'm by no means an expert at teaching sexual health to kids with special needs, but luckily I have colleagues who are. I also have friends who parent kids with special needs. Using their combined invaluable insights, I've compiled what I think are useful, concrete tips on how to empower your child or teen with sexual health and safety information.

A note before we start: I hope my decision to use the term "special needs" to refer to a multitude of developmental differences and delays doesn't seem too general or simplistic. I fully recognize that every child and teen has unique experiences, challenges, and needs, and I want to honour those. I also know that some kids have a dual diagnosis that complicates how they learn and process information. So as you read, please know that my intent isn't to generalize, but to offer guidance to the widest possible range of parents.

I also want to take a moment to congratulate you. If you're having a tough time thinking of your child as a sexual being because of their special needs, you're not alone. And if you're thinking, "We already have enough challenges to contend with, now we have to deal with sex education, too?!" I don't blame you one bit. But I know you can do this. You've already shown how brave you are just by starting to read this chapter. Let's take it one step at a time, together.

In consulting with my colleagues Margaret Newbury Jones and Jessica Wollen, sexual health educators who specialize in teaching sexual health to kids with special needs, I was pleased to find that we're on the same page when it comes to key factors that need to be considered.

First, the more we are open with our kids (regardless of their abilities), the more we're setting them up for safe, healthy, happy relationships in their adult life. As parents, we need to establish ourselves early

> My brother is autistic. Does he need to know this too?

on as our kids' number one source of sexual health information, and this includes teaching our values and beliefs. Especially for kids with special needs, *not* talking sends a message that sexual feelings and relationships aren't allowed. This may lead to our kids hiding both healthy and potentially dangerous behaviours, not to mention feelings of shame and guilt. You know how to best connect with your child. This chapter can offer tips, like I said, but you're the expert.

"Being open" means we need to teach young people with special needs the same information we teach typical kids. And all of the good practices we use with typical kids are good practice for those with special needs. For example, we need to give them information even if they aren't asking questions. When they *do* ask questions, we need to take them seriously and answer honestly. We need to take advantage of every teaching opportunity and we need to talk about sexual health in an open, positive, and light-hearted way. And, recognizing that all kids differ in their learning styles, we need to provide information using a variety of methods.

Second, we need to acknowledge the tragic reality that kids with special needs are especially vulnerable to sexual abuse. Indeed, www.sexualityandu.ca reports that as many as 80% of girls who have special needs and 50% of boys who have special needs will be sexually abused before the age of 18. And, as in the general population, the majority of this abuse is perpetrated by those known to the victim, such as a caregiver or peer. This means that safety information needs to go beyond stranger danger. Teaching kids ownership of their body is critical, as is teaching the skills and language to report an exploitative situation.

Third, although many people view special needs kids as perpetually childlike and asexual, sexual development is almost always the same in kids with special needs as it is in typical kids. Unless they have a particular syndrome and your doctor or specialist has told you about any differences in your child, expect that they'll go through puberty, be fertile, and experience sexual attraction in much the same way as their peers do. They also have the same sexual needs and desires as typical teens and adults, and eventually will want to have romantic relationships. In fact, 60% to 90% of people with mild disabilities report wanting to marry and have children in the future (www.sexualityandu.ca).

With those factors in mind, here are some teaching tips I hope can guide you as you start an ongoing sexual health conversation with your child or teen.

■ ELEMENTARY-AGED CHILDREN

Don't wait for a crisis to start teaching your child about sexual health and safety. Children, especially those with special needs, need preventative information and skills to deal with potentially exploitative or embarrassing situations. Be proactive so that your child feels prepared to handle difficult situations even when you aren't around. Whenever possible, use visuals to reinforce these concepts and messages.

From day one, be a good role model. Our kids listen to everything we say and watch everything we do. Knowing that, we can teach about the important concepts of public and private without even saying a word. Make sure the door is closed when you're going to the bathroom. Don't walk in on other family members when they're in the bathroom. Ask for privacy when you're showering. Change your baby's diaper in private and, although I wholeheartedly support breastfeeding in public, consider doing this in private as well. As you can imagine, seeing a woman reveal (even some of) her breast in public can be very confusing, if a child has just learned that breasts are a private part of the body.

Once you've modelled it, talk and teach explicitly about the difference between public and private. This sets the stage for future discussions about bodies, safety, and social skills. When we're alone in our

> *Can people with special needs get married.*

bedroom or bathroom at home, that's private. Talking with a doctor or a nurse or other medical professional is also private. But school is public. Give clear examples of what we talk about in private versus what we talk about in public. We only talk about bodies, for example, in private. The only exception to this rule is in the classroom with an adult present. This can be confusing, so give clear examples of when and where it's appropriate to learn and talk about sexual health. It wouldn't be a good idea to share your sexual feelings with people on the playground at recess, because the playground is a public space.

Identify the three private parts on the body: the mouth, breasts, and genitals. Stress to your child that it's not appropriate to show private body parts to other people, especially in public. It's also not okay for someone to go on their private parts without their permission. Because much of the abuse of kids with special needs involves grooming victims to touch a perpetrator's body, it's equally important to teach refusal skills.

Teach your child ownership of their body, the idea that they say who goes on them or who touches them and who doesn't. Stress that no one has a right to go on their private parts without their permission, not even a parent or caregiver. If someone does, they need to get away as soon as possible. Practice saying "No" or "Stop" in a strong, bossy voice, or using body language to convey the message. If your child is verbal, teach and repeat key phrases such as, "My body belongs to me," "I'm the boss of my body," and "I don't like that." And if they're in a situation and saying those things doesn't work, teach them they're allowed to use their body to get away.

To reinforce these messages, respect your child's need for privacy. If possible, when they're changing, toileting, and bathing, ask if they'd like you to leave and check in again in a few minutes. If they make comments about you always being naked in front of them, take that cue to close the door when you're changing. Teach words like "dressed" and "undressed" and talk about them in relation to public and private. Use pictures to illustrate this, if helpful.

Use scientific words for body parts. If your child uses an augmentative or alternative communication (AAC) device, make sure that this language is available to them on their device. If your child communicates using American Sign Language (ASL), teach the signs explicitly. Discourage the use of slang, because it's important, particularly for kids with special needs, to have the language they need to report sexual abuse. Having said that, we encourage parents to teach their high-functioning kids the meaning of common slang words. This is to help them avoid repeating the slang they hear other kids use, thinking it's cool.

Use concrete examples. If an aide is helping them with toileting, it's appropriate that they might see or even touch their genitals. Or, if a caregiver is helping them to change their clothes, they may see their breasts. But if they went to the doctor because they had a sore throat, it wouldn't be appropriate to take off their jeans. Whenever and wherever possible, use visuals to reinforce messages. Act it out, draw a picture, use photos from the Internet.

Teach the importance of reporting abuse to a trusted adult, even if the abusive person is someone they know, and practice what to say when reporting. If the first person they tell doesn't take them seriously or help them right away, they need to keep reporting until someone does help them. And someone *will* help them. If your child is nonverbal, provide them with pictures they can use to communicate exploitative touching to an adult. Remember that most kids with special needs don't disclose abuse verbally. Rather, they use changes in behaviour, such as refusing to go with a particular person or refusing to bathe, to communicate it. Because these behaviours can easily be interpreted as acting out, be mindful not to dismiss them.

Teach and model healthy boundaries. Give examples from their own life of appropriate and inappropriate behaviour in social situations. Learning about giving physical affection is a big one. Ask, **"Would it be appropriate to kiss or hug someone you don't know?" "Would it be okay for a person to kiss or hug their boss at work?" "Does it make sense to give someone a hug for no reason?" and "How can you tell if someone doesn't want to be hugged?"** We tend to teach children with developmental differences to be compliant, which is why they're at increased risk for abuse. But this also means that if healthy boundaries are taught in a way they understand, they're more likely to follow them than typical kids. Even if a child is non-verbal, we can gently guide an inappropriate kiss, for example, into an appropriate hug or handshake. Part of this teaching involves asking friends and family members to ask permission before hugging and kissing your child. Grandma may be a bit put off at first, but explain that your request is necessary for your child to maintain healthy boundaries and stay safe. Hopefully she'll understand.

Establish proper procedures for toileting at school. Children with special needs always have a right to know who's going to be helping them and what that will look like. For example, latex gloves should always be used and, if possible, children should learn to wipe themselves (they can do this by placing their hand inside the hand of the care provider who's guiding them). If the person who usually helps them with toileting is away, let your child know ahead of time who will be filling in. In a perfect world, there would be three school staff members known to your child who have been trained to do this work. These people would be specified in your child's Individualized Education Program (IEP). A substitute teacher should never toilet a child; allowing this teaches your child that it's okay for a stranger to touch their body.

Recognizing that people with special needs are sexual beings and have many of the same sexual feelings as typical kids and adults, teach your child about masturbation. Visual aids available on sexual health websites such as www.shift-education.com may be helpful for this.

Specify that it's only appropriate to masturbate when they're alone in their bedroom with the door and curtains closed. Some parents even refer to masturbation as "bedroom behavior." Allow private time in their bedroom or on a regular basis. Stress that it would be not only inappropriate, but also illegal to masturbate in a public place. There's an unfair assumption that children and teens with special needs aren't able to understand or control their sexual feelings and urges. Even worse, some adults hesitate to teach them about masturbation thinking that it will "give them ideas." These assumptions simply aren't true; they stem from ignorance.

Much like typical children, some children with special needs don't understand or are dismayed by the changes to their bodies during puberty. This is especially difficult for children who may not have the communication skills needed to verbalize their concerns. Talk about puberty as a normal and healthy part of growing up and use pictures to demonstrate how everyone's body changes over time. To be concrete, discuss specifically how their body is changing. They may not notice that their peers are going through puberty, too, so make sure to point this out. Stress that everyone in the world goes through puberty, but all bodies develop at different rates. This is a good thing because it makes us all unique!

Besides physical changes, don't forget that, in much the same way as typical kids, kids with special needs will experience emotional changes, like mood swings, during puberty. Recognize and celebrate these changes as normal and explain them to your child as best you can.

Remember that comprehensive sexual health education isn't just about sex. Depending on their level of understanding, teach relationship and sexual values just like you would a typical child. Your child also needs information and skills when it comes to communication, relationships, and boundaries. Point out healthy relationships, and give firm guidelines around when it's appropriate for a first kiss, dating, and a romantic or sexual relationship. Use visuals like TV shows, movies, or what you see around you to illustrate these healthy boundaries.

Keep care providers, school staff, and close relatives in the loop. Let them know what you've been teaching your child, and encourage them to reinforce these positive messages using a common language and consistency. If students are learning about body science in the classroom, make sure it's specified in your child's IEP that someone will review the material with them after. Ideally, they would do this using a different teaching method than was used in class to increase understanding.

Go slower than slow, repeat and review. Repeat and review again. Give your child extra time to process new information, and don't teach anything new until you're sure they have a good grasp of the last concept you taught. If your child is a non-reader, use pictures and read body science books to them as much as possible.

Kids with special needs may be confused by what they've heard from their friends, especially slang words. Many also have difficulty with abstract concepts like relationships and privacy, meaning they have trouble visualizing and seeing pictures in their heads in the same way that others may be able to do. When they listen to someone speak, they can often repeat very accurately what they've heard, but may not fully understand. Knowing this, we need to teach the same concepts in different ways. We can also use TV shows, movies, and real-life situations to illustrate concepts. Ask lots of questions to confirm their understanding.

Just as we do when teaching typical kids, go with what interests your child. If your child likes picture books, use them. If they prefer you to read a book to them, go with that. Explore educational websites or apps if they enjoy going online. Keep it interesting. Be creative and try new ways of teaching to make it as engaging and as fun as possible.

■ TEENS

In addition to everything you teach your elementary-aged child about sexual health, here are some tips for helping your teen understand and enjoy healthy social and romantic relationships as they approach adulthood.

It's totally normal for your teen to experience crushes and sexual attraction to their peers, but they need to be taught appropriate social skills to handle these feelings. Remind them that sexual feelings are healthy, but private. And although they may feel comfortable with everyone knowing who they're crushing on, their crush may not. Respecting boundaries is important.

Foster a community. This isn't just to provide your teen with a social life now, but to offer companionship later in life. Support your teen in setting up times to hang out and socialize with friends outside of school or teen club. Find a like-minded family with a teen of a similar age and get to know them.

Teach conversation skills by practicing a conversation chain. "We're talking about Minecraft right now. What's a question you could ask your friend about Minecraft?" Role-play taking turns asking questions, waiting their turn to answer, and staying on topic.

Ensure that your teen socializes with people of the same age as they are. A teen with special needs playing with a younger child may be a good match intellectually, but could lead to exploitative behaviour. I'm not suggesting for one second that teens with special needs are sexual predators, but that the power imbalance due to the age difference could be problematic. Plus, other people might interpret their behaviour incorrectly. The arousal that's natural during puberty can be confusing for a teen with special needs.

Although your teen's developmental age may be much younger than their chronological age, avoid over-emphasizing it. If a 14-year-old is constantly compared to an eight-year-old, for example, they'll never be viewed by others as a maturing teen. Treating them as much as possible as their same-age peers, on the other hand, helps them to develop emotional maturity and age-appropriate social behaviour. It also honours the 14 years of life experience they have under their belt!

Romantic relationships are not only possible in the teen years, but can be healthy too. Provide guidelines around who they can be in a relationship with. For example, your teen and the other person need to be within a certain number of years in age. Although your teen may feel sexual attraction to someone much younger than they are, because that's where they are intellectually, these feelings may not be appropriate. If feelings are mutual and both teens would like to be in a relationship (which is not always the case), don't discourage it. Chaperone movie dates, provide opportunities for them to spend alone time together, invite your teen's partner to spend time with *your* family, and communicate openly with *their* parent(s).

Teach relationship manners and rules. Talk to your teen how to be a respectful partner. Again, give concrete, literal guidelines. For example, **"You have to go on ten dates before a first kiss." "Always ask before giving your partner a hug." "If you got to choose the last movie you saw together, let them choose the next one."** Don't forget to teach phone and online relationship etiquette, too. It's not out of the question for a teen with special needs to call or text a romantic interest 50 to 60 times a day. Use concrete examples such as, **"You can text your friend five times per day, but if they're not answering you, then it's rude to continue."**

Speaking of the Internet, ensure that you monitor your teen's online activity and presence in much the same way you would with a typical child. We can't assume that just because a teen can't read well or isn't verbal they can't access pornography, inappropriate websites, and chat rooms. Without an understanding of healthy boundaries and general safety online, your child is at risk for exploitation.

If your teen has special needs and is in a sexual relationship, conversations about contraception are just as important as for typical teens. Explicit guidelines as to where they can have sex are also key, as are the basics of sexual consent (in and outside the context of a relationship). Teach them that sexual consent involves an enthusiastic "Yes." Not saying "No" doesn't mean "Yes." Even if they *do* consent to sexual activity, they can change their mind at any time. Let them know that sexual contact without consent is illegal. Using contraception may prevent pregnancy, but it doesn't prevent the trauma of sexual abuse.

Ensure that your teen gets the same sexual health care that typical teens receive. Ask them if they feel comfortable with their doctor. If not, it might be time to look for a new one. Many hospitals and health care centres have clinics for people with special needs that offer more time with patients and specialized treatment. If your teen has testicles, teach them (or help them) to examine them every month. If your teen has a uterus, make sure they're getting regular Pap smears starting at age 21, or within three years of their first sexual contact. Encourage your teen to tell you about or show you any concerns or changes they notice in their body. Even if they're not sexually active, this is all part of good health care. It's also empowering your teen to take responsibility for their body.

> **ANSWERS TO COMMON QUESTIONS ASKED BY PARENTS OF KIDS WITH SPECIAL NEEDS**
>
> **I've taught my child that masturbation is normal and healthy, but private. They understand that at home, but what if they do it at school?**
>
> Especially in the younger years, your child will not be the first ever to masturbate at school! Even typical kids need reminders of where and when it is appropriate to do it. If your child doesn't masturbate in common areas of your home, chances are they won't do it at school either. But if it does happen, first make sure there isn't something irritating their genital area. It's also quite common for younger kids to masturbate if they are feeling stressed, overwhelmed, or needing of a break from class activities.
>
> If this isn't the case, establish open communication with the classroom teacher so that you can work together to reinforce the message that masturbation is a bedroom behaviour. Some teachers tell me that having a key word to use with a student, say, when they start to masturbate during circle time, works really well. When they see a student's hand go down the pants, saying the key word is enough to redirect them. A bonus is that classmates don't usually clue in to what the teacher is referring to, so disruption and potential embarrassment is minimal.

I know that kids with special needs are at high risk of being sexually abused. How do I make sure this doesn't happen to my child?

Kids with special needs *are* at greater risk of abuse for many reasons. They're often taught to be passive and obedient and to trust all caregivers (most perpetrators are known to the victim) and they may also lack boundaries and communication skills that help keep them safe. But you're already helping your child protect themselves by teaching about public versus private, ownership of their body, what appropriate behaviour looks like, and how to report. Teaching these concepts also empowers your child to speak up when something feels uncomfortable or when they know that their boundaries aren't being respected.

My child is overly friendly and trusting. What can I do to protect him?

Teaching our kids how to interact appropriately and safely with others is an ongoing process. Especially for kids with special needs, we need to use good role modelling and practice using concrete examples relevant to their lives. Demonstrate for them what appropriate behaviour looks like with different people. Show them how to greet, show affection to, and thank others depending on how well they know the people. There are good resources to help you do this, such as the Circles program for teens and adults (see Resources section below).

I worry about my child respecting privacy and boundaries at school. What if they walk out of the bathroom with their pants down? What if they try to explore someone else's body?

When it comes to exposing their bodies in public, younger kids with special needs often do this because they have difficulty pulling their pants up, or doing up buttons and zippers on their own after toileting. So try to make sure your child wears pants they can pull up and down by themselves.

To confuse matters, boys with special needs are often taught to urinate at home with their pants pulled down around their ankles. So we can't blame them when they do the same thing when they use a urinal at school, or a public washroom. Teaching your child how to use bathroom stalls and urinals is important. For example, leaving an empty urinal between them and another person not only allows privacy, but is also good manners.

Generally, though, if you've taught your child at home (through role modelling, visual aids, and talking) about the private parts of the body and the importance of keeping them private, chances are good they'll apply those rules at school. Review their toileting routine while at school and offer praise, for example, when they pull up their pants before opening the door at home. Remember that kids with special needs often thrive on consistency. If healthy boundaries are taught repeatedly and consistently in a way they understand, they're even more likely to follow them than typical kids! And if your child makes a mistake, oh well. Adults at their school are there to support them in their learning and to reinforce the important messages and habits you're teaching at home.

I've talked to my daughter and have read books with her about puberty and I feel like she generally understands what to expect. But what about when she gets her period? That just seems like too much for her to handle!

Kudos to this parent for being proactive and teaching her daughter about puberty before she is in the thick of it. Her understanding of her changing body will definitely help her adjust as she matures. Talking openly about puberty will also help her understand how her peers are developing. This may avoid or lessen the possibility that she'll ask her friends inappropriate questions. When it comes to periods specifically, emphasize what a healthy and normal part of growing up it is to have them. Show pictures to explain what happens during a period, and talk about how she'll need to wear something to catch the drips as they come out each month.

If you're comfortable (and you menstruate), bring her into the bathroom when you're changing a pad. Methodically explain what you're doing as you do it, including proper disposal. If you'd prefer, you could demonstrate pad use by putting a pad in underwear and using a mixture of corn starch, water, and food coloring to show how to determine when a pad needs to be changed.

If your daughter has help from an aide when toileting at school, talk to both of them about what that role will look like during a period. Give her lots of time to adjust to having a period, especially if her periods are irregular (new skills might be difficult to remember if she's using them only sporadically at first). And don't forget to consider side effects, like cramps, that she may need your help to manage.

How can I help my child make friends?

Encourage your child to participate in activities they enjoy and praise their openness to try new things. Connect with like-minded families who have kids of similar ages and make plans to socialize together. Allow your child to have alone time with their friends, too, even just for short periods of time. If your child is verbal, teach basic conversation skills. For example, practice taking turns asking and answering questions. Teach basic interpersonal skills, like sharing. Siblings can help with this!

Whenever possible, host birthday parties and accept invitations to other people's parties. Identify your child's interests and build those into play-dates or get-togethers with friends. Doing a Lego project or craft together, for example, can increase comfort and help with bonding. Many parents would prefer that their child only interact with typical kids. But it's okay and likely more successful (particularly when they get older) for their kids to socialize with kids who are similar in abilities.

What if my teen with special needs wants to be in a relationship with a typical teen?

When it comes to relationships, your teen may need some guidance around who would be appropriate for them to be in a relationship with. Of course, the person needs to be of a similar chronological age. But developmental age and ability is important, too. Sometimes kids with special needs feel attraction to typical kids because they've grown up in inclusive environments and may not notice their differences. That is, they may not recognize how they're unique and, in many ways, this is a good thing! But we wouldn't want a teen with special needs to be ridiculed or get hurt feelings for showing attraction to a typical teen, if it's not appropriate. Although crushes are totally normal and healthy, we also wouldn't want a teen with special needs to crush on a movie star, for example, to the point that they believe a relationship with them might actually happen.

As much as possible, provide opportunities for socializing with teens who would be appropriate partners. Talk to your teen about what they might look for in a partner and help them identify those characteristics in their peers. I know it sounds a bit like an arranged marriage, but parents play a big role in facilitating healthy relationships for their teens. And, as hard as it is, prepare your teen for the fact that a person they would like to be in a relationship with may not like them back. This is a tough lesson we all need to learn!

As I acknowledged earlier, teaching sexual health to kids with special needs can be daunting, and I don't blame parents one bit for struggling with the mere thought of it. But remember that *you're* the expert at talking to your kids, and you've taken an important first step just by being open to the ideas and suggestions in this chapter. As you start these conversations, try to stay lighthearted. Don't take yourself too seriously. Be patient with yourself and with your child. Learning can be exhausting for kids with special needs, especially when it comes to abstract concepts. Don't expect too much too soon, and don't take it personally if your child is struggling to understand. Try different approaches and keep your eye on the prize – your child growing up to be a safe, empowered, and healthy adult who can enjoy meaningful relationships in a community of support. *Yes!*

RESOURCES

FOR PARENTS

EDUCATORS

▪ Margaret Newbury Jones is a sexual health educator who specializes in teaching kids with intellectual and developmental delays. newburyjones@gmail.com

▪ Jessica Wollen specializes in teaching sexual health education to individuals with intellectual disabilities, and to professionals and families in community with special needs children, youth, and adults. www.shift-education.com

▪ Paula Bentley is an educator who teaches sexual health education to those with diverse learning needs, their support networks, and other professionals. www.paulabentley.ca

▪ Dave Hingsburger is an educator at Vita Community Services in Toronto, Ontario, and author of many books on sexuality and healthy relationships supporting caregivers and individuals with special needs http://diverse-city.com/online-store-2/books/. Read his blog at www.davehingsburger.blogspot.com.

ONLINE LIBRARY

▪ Sunny Hill Health Centre for Children is a facility in Vancouver, British Columbia, that promotes better health for children with disabilities through clinical services, education, and research. They have an extensive online library of resources (books, pamphlets, DVDs) for teaching children and teens with special needs about sexual health. They offer free shipping of materials within the province of British Columbia. http://www.bcchildrens.ca/our-services/sunny-hill-health-centre

TEACHING KITS

▪ *Circles: Intimacy and Relationships – Levels 1 and 2.* This resource is intended for older teens and adults, not young children. It's recommended that parents seek the guidance of a sexual health educator to work through the videos with their kids. This DVD series by Marklyn P. Champagne and Leslie Walker-Hirsch involves categorizing social roles and designating the colour circle with its associated Three "T's": Touch, Talk, and Trust. Video mini-dramas illustrate common social relationships and display typical touching behaviours, as well as conversation levels and degrees of safety. In *Circles*, the emphasis is on matching the social role with the appropriate circle colour and teaching students to model behaviours that are parallel to those seen on the video.

■ *Janet's Got Her Period* and the *Gyn Exam*: both of these are James Stanfield publications and include DVDs and guide books.

■ These teaching kits are available for loan at http://www.bcchildrens.ca/our-services/sunny-hill-health-centre

BOOKS

■ *An Exceptional Children's Guide to Touch: Teaching Social and Physical Boundaries to Kids*, by McKinley Hunter Manasco and Katharine Manasco.

■ *Asperger's Syndrome and Sexuality: From Adolescence through Adulthood*, by Isabelle Hénault.

■ *Autism: I Have Desires Too* and *How to Teach Your Autistic Teen about Sex: Advanced Guidebook for Parents and Educators*, by Travis Breeding.

■ *I Openers: Parents Ask Questions about Sexuality and Children with Developmental Disabilities*, by Dave Hingsburger, published by The Family Support Institute. www.familysupportbc.com

■ *Sexuality: Your Sons and Daughters with Intellectual Disabilities*, by Karin Melberg Schwier and Dave Hingsburger.

■ *Sexuality and Relationship Education for Children and Adolescents with Autism Spectrum Disorders: A Professional's Guide to Understanding, Preventing Issues, Supporting Sexuality and Responding to Inappropriate Behaviours*, by Davida Hartman.

■ *Sexuality and Severe Autism: A Practical Guide for Parents, Caregivers, and Health Educators*, by Kate E. Reynolds.

■ *Teaching Children with Down Syndrome about Their Bodies, Boundaries, and Sexuality*, by Terri Couwenhoven.

FOR CHILDREN AND TEENS

DOCUMENTARY

■ *Monica & David* is a 2009 documentary by Alexandra Codina. The film focuses on the daily lives of Monica and David, a young married couple with Down syndrome. The film premiered on November 22, 2009 at IDFA and won Best Documentary Feature at the 2010 Tribeca Film Festival. *Monica & David* later had a television premiere on HBO on October 14, 2010.

BOOKS

■ *Making Sense of Sex: A Forthright Guide to Puberty, Sex and Relationships for People with Asperger's Syndrome*, by Sarah Atwood.

■ *The Girls' Guide to Growing Up: Choices and Changes in Your Tween Years* and *The Boys' Guide to Growing Up: Choices and Changes During Puberty*, by Terri Couwenhoven.

■ *Things Ellie Likes: A Book about Sexuality and Masturbation for Girls and Young Women with Autism and Related Conditions*, by Kate E. Reynolds.

■ *Things Tom Likes: A Book about Sexuality and Masturbation for Boys and Young Men with Autism and Related Conditions*, by Kate E. Reynolds.

■ *What's Happening to Ellie?: A Book about Puberty for Girls and Young Women with Autism and Related Conditions*, by Kate E. Reynolds.

■ *What's Happening to Tom?: A Book about Puberty for Boys and Young Men with Autism and Related Conditions*, by Kate E. Reynolds.

CONCLUSION

FROM BODY SCIENCE TO SEXUALLY MATURE ADULT

Especially on tough days (like after teaching a class of squirrely, grossed out Grade 5 kids on a hot Friday afternoon in June, or when a parent suggests that I've stolen their child's innocence by telling them the truth about how babies are made), I find myself reflecting on my purpose as a sexual health educator.

What's my goal in giving kids this information, and how will it affect their lives today and in the future? I know that in the short term, learning about healthy bodies and healthy sexuality will reduce their chances of being abused. I also know that it will help them to make smart decisions about their bodies and, therefore, keep them healthy. In the long term, my hope is that learning about sexuality in a positive, comprehensive way will help them to grow up to be sexually mature adults supported by a sexually mature society. I'm sure this means different things to different people, but here are my thoughts on what that would look like.

THE SEXUALLY MATURE ADULT

Sexually mature adults have a respect and understanding for society's laws and boundaries around sexuality. In a sexually mature society, people respect sexuality as a beautiful but private aspect of their lives. They also respect others' need for privacy, and understand and appreciate the importance of healthy boundaries. (Think back to the sexually immature dad watching TV in his underwear, which prevented his daughter from feeling comfortable inviting friends over.)

In terms of respecting the law, a sexually mature person would never share photos online of someone else without their consent. They would also never produce or watch pornography involving children or animals. And it goes without saying that they would never sexually abuse or exploit in their relationships. In the context of community, sexually mature adults oppose sexual injustice and discrimination and encourage others to do so as well.

Sadly, an adult's history of abuse or trauma can prevent them from having healthy relationships themselves. Sexually mature adults recognize this and seek the support they need in order to heal and move forward. They strive to create (HERI) relationships based on **H**onesty, **E**quality, **R**espect, and **I**ntegrity, and encourage their kids through role modelling and lots of conversations to do the same.

A sexually mature adult also understands and appreciates the importance of consent in relationships free of physical and emotional exploitation. They clearly express their boundaries and have the courage to share with their partner what they enjoy and don't enjoy when it comes to sex. They know that the vulnerability this requires will only bring them closer together. In much the same way, they would never engage in sexual activity they weren't absolutely sure their partner was into.

Sexually mature adults love and celebrate their bodies, imperfections and all, at every stage of life. They aren't afraid to explore their bodies or to masturbate, and don't have hang-ups about nudity. Beyond an appreciation for their physical body, they embrace their uniqueness, and value who they are, their special talents and their abilities. With this self-awareness comes the ability to think critically about the images and messages they see in the media. They're able to stand up for themselves, and to live a life that reflects their true selves, regardless of social pressure or gender stereotypes.

Love for one's body leads sexually mature adults to get regular sexual health exams by a doctor. They also do the self-examinations necessary to keep their bodies healthy (for example, regular breast and testicular self-exams). I believe more than ever that if we're teaching our kids to respect their bodies and to take responsibility for their health, we need to set a good example. As sexually mature adults, we do this by regularly monitoring changes in our bodies and by being brave enough to go to our doctor if we notice anything different.

Almost nine years ago, at age 36, I was diagnosed with breast cancer. I found a lump one night and went to the doctor the very next day. Today I'm cancer-free, but I often think about where I'd be now if I hadn't found that lump myself, as I wasn't due for my first mammogram for another four years. And what if I *had* found the lump, but delayed going to my doctor (as many women do) because life got in the way, or I was just plain scared?

Some parents are concerned that I teach Grade 6 and 7 students about testicular cancer and the importance of doing self-exams at least every month. They worry that I'll frighten their kids unnecessarily given the relative unlikelihood that they'll be affected. But I guarantee that my three friends who have beat testicular cancer were grateful they knew about Testicle Tuesday. Awareness doesn't have to be scary.

A sexually mature adult gets information from credible sources and thinks critically about what they hear and see around them. They use this information – along with respect for themselves and others, and their personal values and beliefs – to make sexual decisions they feel proud of. Sexually mature adults understand that we all have rights, responsibilities, and choices in our relationships. They have a clear idea of what their boundaries and beliefs are, but don't judge other people when they make decisions that aren't consistent with their own value system (for example, a devout Catholic who financially supports a program for pregnant and parenting teens).

Regardless of what our personal beliefs are, sexually mature adults understand that every person and every relationship deserves respect. They don't use homophobic or transphobic language and have the courage to stand up and object when others do. In a sexually mature society, differences in gender identity, how we express our gender and sexuality, or who we want to be in a relationship with, are not only accepted, but *celebrated*.

When I'm teaching at elementary schools in Vancouver, it's not unusual for 80% of the students to come from a variety of immigrant cultures. By this I mean that the students themselves were born in another country, or they were born in Canada but their parents or ancestors emigrated from another country. When people from more conservative countries come to North America, they see overt sexuality in everything around them: in TV shows and movies, in commercials being used to sell pretty much anything, in how we talk, in how we dress, and in our seemingly *laissez-faire* attitude toward sex. Not surprisingly, their biggest fear is that we educators are going to tell their kids, "Sex is no big deal," or "Sex is great, have it as much as possible!"

In a sexually mature society, cultural and religious values can still be honoured, especially those that encourage basic human rights and responsibilities. But we can also recognize that traditions of taboo and silence put our children at risk. Sexually mature adults appreciate the protective value of education. They ensure that their kids have the information they need while at the same time teach the values that serve as their moral compass.

Sexually mature adults can share boundaries and guidelines with their kids in a way that's sex positive and sexually mature. Within the context of whatever their family and religious values tell them, they can also teach their kids that sexuality should be celebrated, that there can be beauty and elegance in our sexual interactions with others. There's no need for parents to be ashamed about having sex or for giving positive messages to kids about the joys and pleasures that a sexual relationship provides.

* * *

So that's it. That's what I hope for our kids' future. It's what they deserve. Do we have a long way to go? We sure do. But can we make it happen? Absolutely, and already you are a huge part of that. Every question you answer, every teachable moment you grab, and every conversation you have with your kids brings them, and all of us, closer to sexual maturity. We need to put our own baggage aside and face our fear so that our kids can live safe, happy and healthy lives. If you ask me, there's no better reason to *talk sex today*.

INDEX

"69", 196, 275

abortion, 106, 256
abuse, 97, 308
    prevention, 47, 87
    reporting, 48
    sex education and, 25–27
adoption, 61, 98, 256
adults with special needs
    sex and, 274
ageism, 100
amniotic sac, 64
anus, 59, 60
asexuality, 38
assertiveness skills, 101

bathing
    nudity and, 274
bathroom humour, 28, 77–79
biological sex, 35
    intersex, 35
birth, 64
bisexual, 38
blow jobs, 194, 275
body image, 121–25, 308
    weight gain at puberty, 121
boundaries, 307, 308
    for intermediates, 98, 101
    for teens, 224
    teaching
        children and teens with special needs, 294, 300
breast
    develop in pubertal boys, 108
    development, 108
    medical examinations, 261
    self-examination, 211, 308
bullying, 126–28, 183
    cyber, 159–63

celibacy, 38
cervical cancer, 259
cervix, 259, 261
Cesarean, 64, 84
checklists
    adolescents, 265
children and teens with special needs
    abuse of, 291
        preventing, 291, 292, 299
    Circles program, 300
    friendships, 302
circumcision, 56
clitoris, 60
condoms, 66, 205, 249–51
    effectiveness, 249
    internal, 250, 251, 255
    rates of use, 203
    safety, 65
    STIs, 104
    STIs and, 250
consent, 243, 244, 308
    Canadian Law, 179
    for preschoolers, 48
    posting and sharing images, 163, 164, 163–64, 175
    teaching, 176
    teens with special needs, 298
consent rules, 178
contraception, 240, 248–55
    condoms, 205, 249
    contraceptive patch, 255
    emergency contraception (EC), 205, 206, 256
    internal condoms, 250
    intrauterine system (IUS), 254
    oral, 251–53
        effectiveness, 251
        STIs and, 252

teens with special needs, 298
vaginal ring, 255
withdrawal method, 253

dating, 193
dildos, 277
double standard, 241–42
dress, 231–34
    inappropriate, 97

emotions
    sads, glads, and mads, 115
equality, 192, 201
erections, 83
    practice, 53, 54–56, 83
exercise, 118

families
    celebrating, 99
    celebrating every kind, 61
family values
    celebrating sexuality, 310
    teaching your, 14, 22, 23, 62, 219
fingering. *See* digital sex
foreskin, 56
    smegma, 59

gender
    stereotypes, 50–51, 122
        Blue box, 180–85
        consent and, 180–82
        Pink Box, 180
gender expression, 34
gender identity, 33, 105, 278
    agender, 33
    cisgender, 37
    discrimination, 36
    gender binary, 33
    genderqueer, 33, 278
    transgender, 35
    third-gender, 33
Genderbread Person, 32
G-spot, 285

HERI (Honesty, Equality, Respect, and Integrity), 192, 193, 201, 308
hermaphrodite. *See* intersex
homophobia, 87, 99, 100, 280
homosexual, 38
honesty, 21, 23, 24, 45, 46, 70, 89, 192, 201, 221, 273
    children and teens with special needs, 290
hygiene, 83, 111, 112
hymen
    virginity and the, 197
hypersexualization, 122, 148

iGirl, 192
iGuy, 180
illustrations
    Genderbread Person, 32
    Bodies with a Penis and Testicles, 55
    Bodies with a Vulva, Vagina, and Clitoris, 60
in vitro fertilization, 62
in vitro fertilization (IVF), 98, 99
inclusivity, 99
integrity, 192, 201
Internet, 101
intersex, 100
    hermaphrodite, 35
    slang terms, 35
intrauterine devices (IUDs), 254–55
    effectiveness, 254
intrauterine insemination (IUI), 98
intrauterine system (IUS), 254

labia, 59
labour, 64
language
    disrespectful, 100, 309
    slang, 100
lesbian, 38
LGBTQ+, 39–40

magical thinking, 45, 61
masturbation, 60, 86, 195, 240, 280, 308

children and teens with special
    needs, 299
  mutual, 195
  teaching privacy, 86
mechanical curiosity, 76
media
  body image, 113, 122, 308
  cyberbullying, 159–63
  distortions of sex, 101, 282
  music, 141–44
  online gaming, 139
  predators, 140
  privacy, 154
  selfies, 158
  setting boundaries and guidelines,
    139
  sexting, 163–67
  smart phones, 155
  social media, 134, 144, 148
  texting dictionary, 156
medical examinations. *See* sexual
    health examinations
menstruation. *See* periods

needles
  safety, 67
nocturnal emissions. *See* wet dreams
nudity, 97, 308
  bathing and, 274
nutrition, 117
  dieting, 117

Options for Sexual Health, 10
orgasms, 60, 283
outercourse, 195
ova, 57
ovaries, 57
  torsions, 58
ovum, 60

Pap smear, 257, 259, 261
parties, 226–31
peer pressure, 241, 242
pelvic exam, 261

penis, 259
  function, 53
  hygiene, 56
  naming, 52
  size, 112
    pornography, 112
periods, 79
  children and teens with special
    needs, 301
  cramps, 113
  cups, 114
  First Period Party, 114
  for intermediates, 113
  for primaries, 81
  pads, 80, 114
  tampons, 81, 114
Planned Parenthood Association of
    British Columbia. *See* Options for
    Sexual Health
pornography, 112, 167–70, 282, 308
power, 182–85
predators, 140
pregnancy, 200, 202, 241, 248, 251
  for intermediates, 105
  miscarriages, 105–6
  myths, 203
  rates, 202
  unplanned, 102, 204–5, 240, 204–5
privacy, 96, 97, 224, 274, 307
  children and teens with special
    needs, 293
  masturbation, 60
  online, 154
  teaching
    children and teens with special
      needs, 291, 300
  teaching about, 24, 47, 85
private parts, 47, 85
  children and teens with special
    needs, 292
puberty
  children and teens with special
    needs, 295

315

**TALK
SEX
TODAY**

for intermediates, 107–20
for primaries, 82
pre-puberty information, 69
pubic hair, 109
    shaving and waxing, 109, 284

racism, 100
rape culture, 179, 181, 182, 183
relationships
    healthy, 219, 241, 243
        definition of, 192
        HERI, 192, 201, 308
    parental, 120
    romantic, 176, 191, 219–23
        as portrayed in media, 191
        social media, 191
        teens with special needs, 296, 298, 302
    unhealthy, 221–22
respect, 192, 201, 309

sads, mads, and glads, 115
scrotum, 57
sensual children, 85
sex
    anal, 195, 198, 275
    celebrating, 63
    cyber or Internet, 195
    digital or manual, 195, 276
    oral, 194, 196, 198, 275
        rates among teens and, 199
        teens and, 241
    phone, 195
    positive messaging, 102, 202, 239, 272, 310
    rates of substance abuse and, 203
    readiness for, 200–201, 244
    vaginal, 194, 196, 198, 240
        rates among teens, 199
        teens and, 241
sex education
    abuse prevention, 25–27
    as cause of experimentation, 21
    benefits, 21, 28, 90

sex toys, 277
sex worker, 279
sexism, 100
sexting, 163–67
sexual activity, 21
    teens and, 198–200, 240–45
sexual arousal, 60
    in children, 60
sexual assault
    emergency contraception, 206
sexual attraction, 38, 202, 219, 240, 279
    homosexual, 38
    lesbian, 38
sexual health examinations, 257–64
sexual health exams, 308
    people assigned female, 259
    people assigned male, 258
sexual intercourse, 62, 98, 101, 194, 284
sexual orientation. See sexual attraction
sexual relationship
    emotional aspects, 102, 201
sexually transmitted infections
    for intermediates, 102–5
    myths, 245–48
sexually transmitted infections (STIs), 200, 202, 207–10, 241, 251, 259, 261, 276
    condoms and, 206
slang, 35, 52, 87, 100
    children and teens with special needs, 293
    hooker, 278
    sexual
        defining for children, 196–97
sleep, 118–20
sleepovers, 225
    parties and, 229
smegma
    foreskin, 59
    vulva, 59
social media. See media
sperm, 58

STDs. *See* sexually transmitted infections (STIs)
stereotypes, 99
   gender, 35, 100, 122
      consent and, 180–82
stool, 59, 60
   sample, 59
suicide, 280
sweat, 111

teens
   pregnancy, abortion, birth rates, 12
   rates of sexual activity, 12
testicles, 57
   function, 58
   medical examinations, 257, 259
   self-examination, 210, 280
   torsions, 58
testicular
   self-examination, 308
testicular cancer, 210
testosterone, 58
tips for talking
   to intermediates, 213
   to preschoolers, 70
   to primaries. *See* tips for talking to preschoolers
   to teens, 262

transgender, 35, 100, 277
   discrimination, 36
transphobia, 100, 280
transsexual, 35
transvestite, 40
twins, 83
   fraternal and identical, 84
   umbilical cords, 84

umbilical cord, 64
urethra
   female, 60
   male, 58
uterus, 63, 259

vagina, 60
   naming, 52, 59
values. *See* family values
vibrators, 240, 277
virginity, 197–98, 281
voice changes, 109
vulva, 52, 59
   hygiene, 113
   smegma, 59

wet dreams, 81, 107

■ SALEEMA NOON, B.A, M.A., O.B.C.

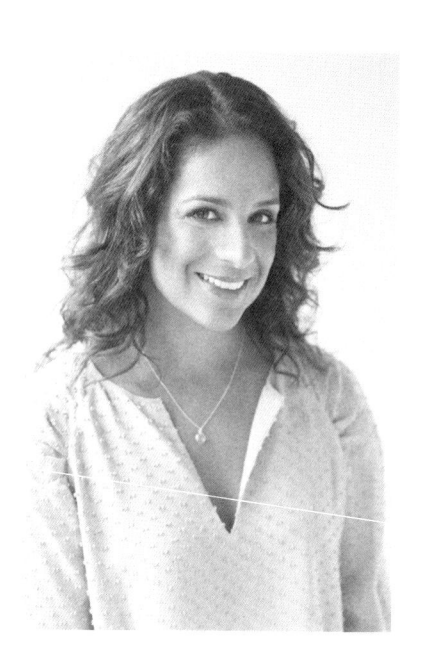

Saleema Noon earned her Bachelor of Arts degree in Family Sciences at UBC. She then researched the quality of sexual health education in B.C. high schools, earning her a Master of Arts degree in sexual health education in 1997, also from UBC. Since then, Saleema has been teaching not only in the field of sexual health, but also in the areas of assertiveness training, Internet safety, healthy relationships, body image and self-esteem. Stepmom to two teenaged girls, she is the creator of the popular iGirl and iGuy Empowerment Workshops for 9–12 year olds.

Respected by the media as a sexual health expert, Saleema has appeared as a regular guest on CTV *Morning Live*, Global News, CBC Radio, CKNW Radio, Shaw TV, CityTV *Breakfast Television* and the *Kid Carson Show* on KISS Radio, and was featured in the CBC Documentary *Sext Up Kids*. Saleema has been featured in *Canadian Living*, *Chatelaine* and *Today's Parent* magazines along with several other national publications, and is the recipient of the Options for Sexual Health's Educator of the Year Award. In 2011, Saleema also received the YWCA Vancouver's Women of Distinction Connecting the Community Award. She is a member of the Order of British Columbia.

MEG HICKLING, C.M., O.B.C, LL.D

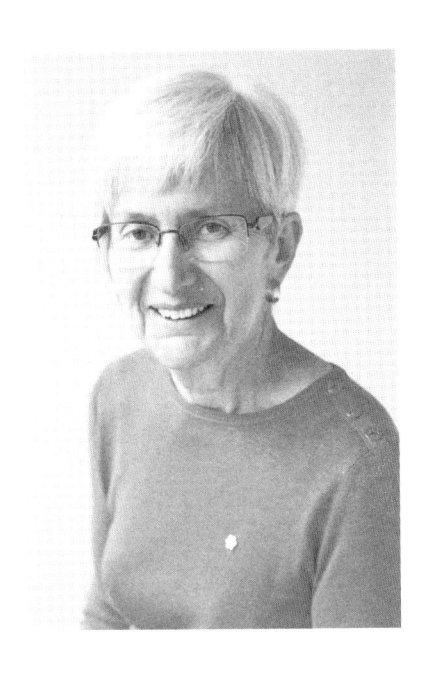

Meg Hickling is a retired registered nurse and an award-winning educator and author who has been instilling knowledge of sexual health in children and adults for over 30 years. Often volunteering her time, she is British Columbia's leading advocate in educating children about human reproduction. Meg believes that knowledge brings about empowerment. Sensitive to her young audiences and their parents, she delivers her message on sexuality and abuse prevention with empathy and a gentle humour. Her ability to convey difficult and controversial material with sensitivity and warmth distinguishes her as a remarkable teacher and role model.

Meg's vision and influence have earned her The Canadian Home and School Federation's Health Award, The YWCA Woman of Distinction Award for Health Education, The RNABC Award of Excellence, and The Distinguished Service to Families Award. In 1997 Meg received The Order of British Columbia and was most notably awarded The Order of Canada in 2000. She is the author of *Meg Hicklings Grown-up Sex: Sexual Wellness for the Better Part of Your Life* (2008, Northstone), *Boys, Girls & Body Science: A First Book about Facts of Life* (2002, Harbour Publishing), and *The New Speaking of Sex* (2005, Northstone).

WOODLAKE

IMAGINING, LIVING, AND TELLING THE FAITH STORY.

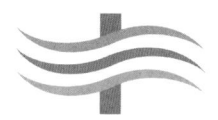

WOOD LAKE IS THE FAITH STORY COMPANY.

It has told
- the story of the seasons of the earth, the people of God, and the place and purpose of faith in the world;
- the story of the faith journey, from birth to death;
- the story of Jesus and the churches that carry his message.

Wood Lake has been telling stories for more than 30 years. During that time, it has given form and substance to the words, songs, pictures, and ideas of hundreds of storytellers.

Those stories have taken a multitude of forms – parables, poems, drawings, prayers, epiphanies, songs, books, paintings, hymns, curricula – all driven by a common mission of serving those on the faith journey.